BASIC CHILD HEALTH: PRACTICE PAPERS

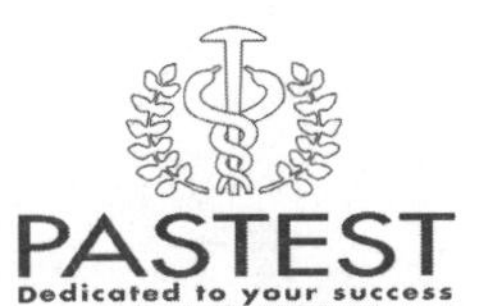

BASIC CHILD HEALTH: PRACTICE PAPERS

Dr Peter de Halpert
MBBS (London) MRCPCH
Specialist Registrar in Paediatrics
Barnet Hospital
Barnet and Chase Farm Hospitals NHS Trust
Barnet, Herts

Dr Ian Pollock
MBBS MRCP FRCPCH DCH DRCOG
Consultant Paediatrician
Chase Farm Hospital
Barnet and Chase Farm Hospitals NHS Trust
Enfield, Middlesex

Dr Jacqueline A Lynch
MBBS MRCS (A&E) DCH DRCOG DIMC
Specialist Registrar
Emergency Medicine
Wessex Deanery

DCH CLINICAL SECTION BY

Dr R M Beattie
BSc MBBS MRCP FRCPCH
Consultant Paediatric Gastroenterologist
Paediatric Medical Unit
Southampton General Hospital
Southampton, Hampshire

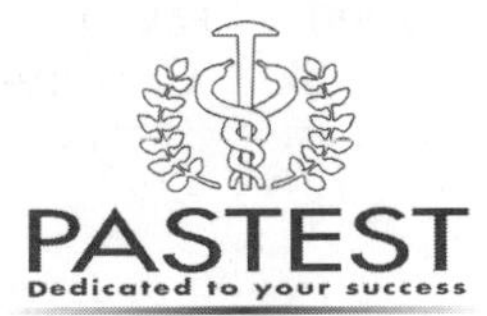

© 2004 PasTest Ltd
Egerton Court
Parkgate Estate
Knutsford
Cheshire, WA16 8DX

Telephone: 01565 752000

First edition 2004

ISBN: 1 904627 080

A catalogue record for this book is available from the British Library.

Typeset by Breeze Ltd, Manchester
Printed by Page Bros, Norwich

CONTENTS

The Clinical Examination

ACKNOWLEDGEMENTS

Dr Jacqueline Lynch wrote the original *Practice Papers for the DCH Examination*. Edited by Dr Ian Pollock and published in 2000, the book quickly became recognised as an essential aid for preparation for the DCH written paper. The Multiple Choice Questions (and their explanations) written by Dr Lynch for the original book remain excellent examples, and have been included in this book, although some have been updated.

I would like to thank all my colleagues who acted as guinea-pigs and were subjected to many questions – their patience and constructive comments are gratefully appreciated.

I would like to dedicate this book to Sarah.

Peter de Halpert

This book is for Joseph

Ian Pollock

I would like to thank all my family and friends for their help with this publication, particularly my parents and I would like to dedicate this book to Niall, Barry, Jamie and of course Rhoderick.

Jacqueline A Lynch

NOTES ON PASSING THE BASIC CHILD HEALTH EXAM

The Diploma of Child Health (DCH) examination is run by the Royal College of Paediatrics and Child Health. It is designed to give recognition of competence in the care of children to general practitioner vocational trainees, staff grades and senior house officers in paediatrics and trainees in specialties allied to paediatrics. The aim is to test knowledge of primary care paediatrics, especially from the following aspects: epidemiology, prenatal care, nutrition and feeding, growth and development, immunisation and screening, health surveillance and promotion, accident prevention, child abuse and legislation, as well as the diagnosis and management of the principal childhood conditions.

THE EXAMINATION

Candidates are advised to have completed a minimum of six months work experience in Paediatrics and Child Health before sitting the examination, as it is unlikely that a candidate would be successful without this experience. The examination consists of two sections:

Written Section – Basic Child Health (Paper One A):

- 40–45 True/false Multiple Choice Questions
- 7–9 Extended Matching Questions
- 17–19 Best of Five Questions

Paper One A will be taken by candidates for the DCH and the Membership of the Royal College of Paediatrics and Child Health (MRCPCH). Candidates for MRCPCH will also have to sit Paper One B (Extended Paediatrics) – these two parts constitute the MRCPCH part 1.

Candidates who have passed either the MRCP (UK) Part 1 examination or Part 1 of the MRCPCH within the previous seven years are exempt from the Written section of the DCH examination.

Clinical Section:

- One Long Case – 40 minutes with the patient and 20 minutes of discussion.
- Short Cases – 30 minutes total of which 10 minutes will be devoted to developmental testing, including the testing of vision/hearing.

NB After passing Paper One A candidates are allowed **three** attempts at the clinical section before having to resit the Paper One A. A failure in either the Long or Short Case cannot be compensated by a good performance in the other section and will result in an overall fail in the examination.

THE WRITTEN PAPERS

Multiple Choice Questions

There are 40–45 questions each having five stems which are either 'True' or 'False'. One mark (+) will be awarded for each correct answer, and so a total of five marks is possible for each question. There is NO negative marking so if you do not know the answer it is always worth putting an answer down, as a 'don't know' or no answer at all will not get you any marks. Remember to read each stem carefully and look out for terms such as 'always/never' (generally False) and 'may/can' (generally True). Usually a brief outline is provided of a common condition found in primary care, followed by four or five questions, often interjected with new information as the story unfolds. However, always answer the question at the stage it is posed without the influence of forthcoming information. Although knowledge of medical management is important, the focus is more on the psychosocial aspects of care of the child and his/her family. It is essential to be familiar with the roles of each member of the multidisciplinary team and be able to advise on health education and prevention, etc.

Extended Matching Questions

Ten possible answers are listed followed by three scenarios. A question will ask for the most correct answer from the list (much as in the same way as the Best of Five – see below).

It is worth noting that as these questions test judgement/experience, some clinicians may not necessarily agree with some of the answers given in this book. This is not to say that the answers here are flawed, just that the answers given are correct in our opinion. Candidates are advised that these practice papers should not form the basis of a revision programme – but should be used as a guide to what the actual questions may be like.

It is worth noting that to provide a list of ten possible answers, sometimes some of the answers listed may be slightly esoteric/uncommon. This paper is designed to test what a candidate is likely to have seen in 6–12 months of hospital, community or primary care paediatrics. If a rare or uncommon cause is listed it may well be a possible answer but it is worth considering that it may be less likely as the paper is not designed to test extended paediatrics.

Best of Five Questions

These questions are designed to test experience and judgement. A short statement will be followed by five possible answers, all of which could be right. The candidate must choose the answer that is the most right. Each of these questions is worth four marks.

Again these questions represent our own opinions.

THE CLINICAL EXAMINATION

The Long Case

In the Long Case you have 40 minutes with the patient. Time management is an important skill that can only be gained by frequent practice under exam conditions. Introducing yourself and chatting to the child and parents for a few minutes will be time well spent, as they will be far more friendly and co-operative than if you jump in with frantic questions. Take a full history including antenatal, immunisations, development and the social situation at home and at school. This is traditionally followed by a full examination, although in a potentially fractious toddler take any opportunity to examine the relevant system while the child is still co-operative. Always remember to plot height and weight on the growth chart, check the BP and test the urine.

Give yourself 10 minutes at the end to prepare a summary, a differential diagnosis, and a suitable management plan. If you still have no idea of the diagnosis, ask the parents; they will more than likely tell you and always check with them if there are areas they think are important which you haven't covered. If they are still unforthcoming, remember, knowing the diagnosis is not as important as demonstrating you have tried to find it out in a logical manner. You then have 20 minutes with the examiners, only 5–10 minutes will be spent on your presentation, the remainder usually being spent testing your knowledge of related aspects to the case. Present the relevant positive or negative findings only. Keep it brief and interesting. List your differential diagnoses in order of probability and avoid mentioning rare causes unless you're prepared to discuss them. End confidently with your initial management plan and be ready to expand on it. Don't forget to take something to write with!

The Short Cases

This section lasts 30 minutes. At least 10 minutes will be spent on developmental assessments and you should be fluent at performing the distraction hearing test, various means of testing vision and eliciting which milestones the child has reached.

The examiners will want to get through as many cases as possible; however, avoid the temptation to lunge at the relevant bit without first introducing yourself and telling the parents and child what you intend to do, although don't procrastinate either. Know the features of common syndromes (eg Down's, Turner's, neurofibromatosis, etc) and when asked to examine a particular system always stick to 'inspection, palpation, percussion and auscultation' – my examination of 'the heart' ended with the observation of a thoracotomy scar. Always be tactful when presenting your findings of a child with dysmorphic features and remember to thank them before moving on to the next case.

Again the best way of passing the Short Cases is endless practice. Bring a paediatric stethoscope and although all other necessary equipment should be provided, do bring your own if you're more comfortable using it. Finally, dress smartly without being overbearing; NEVER EVER argue with the examiners and of course – Good Luck!

PAPER 1

MULTIPLE CHOICE QUESTIONS

1.1 Congenital hypertrophic pyloric stenosis

- ○ A has an incidence of 4 per 1000 live births
- ○ B typically presents with projectile bile-stained vomiting
- ○ C is more common in girls
- ○ D may cause hyperkalaemic alkalosis
- ○ E the investigation of choice is an ultrasound scan (USS)

1.2 In children the features of nephrotic syndrome include:

- ○ A Proteinuria, hypoalbuminaemia, generalised oedema and hyperlipidaemia
- ○ B The most common cause of idiopathic (primary) nephrotic syndrome is diffuse proliferative glomerulonephritis
- ○ C Serum albumin < 35 g/l
- ○ D A high protein, no-salt diet should be strictly adhered to
- ○ E A peak incidence of between 2 and 5 years of age

1.3 Regarding low birth weight (LBW) infants:

- ○ A Premature infants are those born before 36 completed weeks' gestation
- ○ B Very low birth weight infants are those weighing < 2500 g
- ○ C There is a characteristic association with maternal diabetes
- ○ D They have an increased incidence of congenital malformations
- ○ E Babies who are small for gestational age (SGA) may reflect maternal diabetes

1.4 Regarding tonsils and adenoids

- A Purulent follicular exudate is present only in bacterial tonsilitis
- B A 3-day course of penicillin is adequate treatment for bacterial tonsillitis
- C Recurrent febrile convulsions associated with attacks of follicular tonsillitis are an indication for tonsillectomy
- D Primary post-tonsillectomy haemorrhage is usually due to infection
- E Adenoidectomy is useful in the treatment of glue ear

1.5 With regard to autism

- A Males and females are equally affected
- B It usually develops after 3 years of age
- C Drugs such as tranquillisers have a role in the management of autism
- D Autistic children commonly have islands of intact intellectual functioning, the so-called idiot savant
- E A diagnosis of autism can be made if the child has two of the following features:
  - global impairment of language and communication
  - impairment of social relationships, especially empathy
  - ritualistic and compulsive phenomena

1.6 In an 8-year-old girl presenting with staining of her underwear and slight yellow discharge at the introitus with no other signs

- A it is urgent to exclude sexual abuse in the first instance
- B vulvovaginitis is the most likely diagnosis
- C *Gardnerella vaginalis* is a common infecting organism
- D lack of labial fat pads protecting the vaginal orifice and the excess acidity of the prepubertal vagina are increased risk factors for infection
- E topical dienestrol cream is a useful treatment

1.7 With regard to blood pressure measurement in children

- ○ A It should be a routine part of cardiovascular examination
- ○ B The correct cuff size is approximately 2/3 the length of the upper arm
- ○ C The 5th Korotkoff sound is used for diastolic measurement
- ○ D Raised blood pressure in children < 6 years is commonly due to primary hypertension
- ○ E A diastolic pressure > 90 mmHg before 13 years requires treatment

1.8 Regarding cot death/near miss cot death

- ○ A If an infant suffers a cot death but their twin appears in excellent health, the parents may be reassured
- ○ B Apnoea monitors do not decrease the incidence of cot death
- ○ C Risk factors include viral infections, prone sleeping position, hypothermia and old polyvinyl chloride (PVC) mattresses
- ○ D Parents should be taught to recognise and assess signs of illness in their babies and be discouraged from frequent visits to the general practitioner (GP) that may result in increased anxiety
- ○ E Parents who stop smoking significantly decrease the risk of their child suffering a cot death

1.9 Regarding acute bronchiolitis

- ○ A Up to 50% of cases are secondary to respiratory syncytial virus (RSV)
- ○ B Nasopharyngeal aspirate may be used for the direct detection of virus in secretions by immunofluorescence
- ○ C Ribavirin is an antiviral agent effective against RSV and should be used as a first-line treatment if RSV infection is confirmed
- ○ D Salbutamol and theophylline have no effect on bronchiolar obstruction under 1 year of age
- ○ E Maternal IgA is protective against RSV

1.10 With regard to eczema

- ○ A In 70% there is a family history of atopy
- ○ B It resolves by 5 years in 80% of children
- ○ C It often starts on the face/neck/behind the ears, but favours extensor surfaces in older children
- ○ D Chinese herbal therapy is of proven benefit in resistant cases
- ○ E Breast-feeding or hypoallergenic formula milk decreases the risk and severity in infants with a positive family history of atopy

1.11 Regarding school refusal

- ○ A It is most common in children aged 11–14 years
- ○ B Children typically come from social classes I and II
- ○ C It is more common in girls
- ○ D It commonly presents with recurrent abdominal pains or headaches
- ○ E It typically occurs in a conscientious and intelligent student

1.12 Causes of persistent snoring in children include:

- ◯ A Hypertrophic nasal turbinates
- ◯ B Hyperthyroidism
- ◯ C Obesity
- ◯ D Down's syndrome
- ◯ E Recurrent tonsillitis

1.13 With regard to oesophageal atresia (OA)

- ◯ A 85% of affected babies will have a tracheo-oesophageal fistula
- ◯ B It may be associated with cardiovascular and urogenital anomalies
- ◯ C Mothers often have oligohydramnios antenatally
- ◯ D It can present with recurrent pneumonia
- ◯ E It is diagnosed by a barium swallow

1.14 With regard to reflexes

- ◯ A The Moro reflex persists from birth to about 3 months
- ◯ B The rooting/suckling and swallowing reflex is usually absent before 34/40
- ◯ C An absent red reflex may indicate a retinoblastoma
- ◯ D The grasping reflex persists from birth to about 3 months
- ◯ E The stepping reflex persists from birth to about 6 months

1.15 Treatment of cystic fibrosis includes:

- ◯ A Regular physiotherapy
- ◯ B Heart and lung transplant
- ◯ C Long-term prophylactic amoxicillin
- ◯ D High-protein, low-fat diet
- ◯ E Pancreatic enzyme supplements with main meals only

1.16 Regarding screening criteria

- A A screening test should have low sensitivity and specificity
- B Acceptable screening tests should give a yield of at least 1 in 100, 000
- C Screening tests should be inexpensive
- D Effective screening tests are available for the majority of conditions
- E Screening must be a continuous process

1.17 Features of a headache that would alert you to the diagnoses of serious intracranial pathology are

- A transient ataxia, hemiparesis or aphasia
- B recent onset of a squint
- C if it wakens the child at night and is most severe first thing in the morning
- D relief on implementing an 'exclusion diet' (ie chocolate, cheese, milk, etc)
- E deterioration in school performance

1.18 Causes of short stature include:

- A Noonan's syndrome
- B Soto's syndrome
- C Turner's syndrome
- D Klinefelter's syndrome
- E Marfan's syndrome

1.19 Conditions that may result in a false-positive sweat test include:

- A Addison's disease
- B Hypothyroidism
- C Diabetes mellitus
- D Nephrogenic diabetes insipidus
- E Bronchiectasis

1.20 The Education Act 1993

- ○ A defines a child with special educational needs (SEN) as one who has a learning difficulty that requires special educational provision to be made
- ○ B states that children whose language of the home is different from the one in which they will be taught may be considered to have a learning difficulty
- ○ C states that children with SEN should be taught in special schools
- ○ D requires a statement of SEN to be made and reviewed regularly
- ○ E states that special educational provision includes any educational provision given to a child under 2 years of age

1.21 Concerning accidents

- ○ A They are the single largest cause of death in children between 1 and 14 years
- ○ B 60% of all childhood deaths are due to accidents
- ○ C The most common fatal accidents are due to falls
- ○ D Approximately 15% of all children per year attend A&E because of an accidental injury
- ○ E The incidence is similar in boys and girls

1.22 Regarding bilirubin toxicity

- A It is caused by free unconjugated bilirubin, which is lipid soluble and therefore readily diffuses across brain cell membranes
- B Kernicterus only occurs when the serum bilirubin exceeds 380 mmol/l
- C The symptoms include hypotonia and lethargy
- D If the baby survives, long-term sequelae include choreoathetoid cerebral palsy and high-frequency nerve deafness
- E Phototherapy uses a narrow spectrum blue light of wavelength 450–475 nm

1.23 The following drugs are safe in breast-feeding:

- A Thyroxine
- B Digoxin
- C Nitrazepam
- D Cimetidine
- E Chlorpheniramine

1.24 Common causes of epistaxis in children include:

- A Nose picking
- B Hypertension
- C Upper respiratory tract infection
- D Atrophic rhinitis
- E Foreign bodies

1.25 Concerning dentition

- ◯ A There are 32 deciduous teeth
- ◯ B Teething causes fever, irritability and excessive salivation
- ◯ C Children do not have the hand-eye co-ordination to adequately clean their teeth until approximately 8–10 years of age
- ◯ D The first tooth to appear is generally a lower central incisor
- ◯ E Malocclusion may result from thumb sucking

1.26 Regarding urinary tract infection (UTI)

- ◯ A It may present with vomiting, irritability and feeding problems
- ◯ B It should be investigated during or after the child's second UTI
- ◯ C Urine specimens can be stored at 0–4 °C for up to 24 hours
- ◯ D The presence of pyuria proves a UTI
- ◯ E Obesity predisposes to UTI in girls

1.27 Regarding scabies

- ◯ A It is caused by the *Sarcoptes scabiei* mite
- ◯ B Burrows usually involve the interdigital webs or flexor aspects of the wrists, while sparing the face and scalps of infants
- ◯ C Symptomatic family members only need to be treated
- ◯ D Itching is usually worse at night
- ◯ E Persistent pruritus 2 weeks later implies failure of treatment

1.28 Regarding obesity

- A It is associated with growth hormone deficiency
- B It may be complicated by Blount's disease
- C It is associated with Lawrence–Moon–Biedl syndrome
- D Most obese healthy children are tall for their age
- E It is associated with hyperparathyroidism

1.29 Management of epilepsy includes:

- A Ketogenic diet
- B Discouraging swimming
- C Wearing protective helmets while cycling alone on open roads
- D Surgery
- E Education in normal schools

1.30 Causes of constipation include:

- A Congenital absence of intestinal autonomic ganglion cells of the Auerbach and Messier plexus
- B Dehydration
- C Hypocalcaemia
- D Hypothyroidism
- E Over-enthusiastic potty training

1.31 Phenylketonuria

- A is an autosomal dominant condition
- B is associated with infantile spasms
- C is detected using the Guthrie test at approximately day 6
- D will result in mental disability if the diagnosis is delayed
- E may harm normal infants in utero if their affected mothers do not maintain their dietary restrictions throughout the pregnancy

1.32 The following are notifiable diseases:

- ○ A Acquired immune deficiency syndrome (AIDS)
- ○ B Mumps
- ○ C Tuberculosis (TB)
- ○ D Rubella
- ○ E Malaria

1.33 Regarding acute lymphoblastic leukaemia (ALL)

- ○ A It accounts for 85% of all childhood leukaemia
- ○ B It commonly presents with bone and joint pain
- ○ C It is more common in girls
- ○ D The presence of a B cell immunological surface membrane marker is associated with the best prognosis
- ○ E Epstein–Barr virus is associated with an increased risk of developing leukaemia

1.34 With regard to spina bifida

- ○ A Spina bifida occulta is seen in 5–10% of all children's spines
- ○ B Arnold–Chiari malformation is frequently associated with myelomeningocele
- ○ C Myelomeningocele characteristically causes spastic paraplegia of the lower limbs
- ○ D Meningocele has no neurological involvement
- ○ E Myelomeningocele is characteristically associated with incontinence of urine, but not of faeces

1.35 Which of the following incubation periods are correct?

- ○ A Chickenpox: 2–5 days
- ○ B Measles: 7–14 days
- ○ C Glandular fever: 14–21 days
- ○ D Mumps: 12–31 days
- ○ E Rubella: 7–14 days

1.36 With regard to cleft palate

- ○ A It may cause hearing loss
- ○ B All babies with cleft palate should be admitted to the special care baby unit (SCBU) for nasogastric feeding (NG) feeding
- ○ C It should be repaired at 3 months
- ○ D Speech develops normally in approximately 75% of children
- ○ E It is associated with maternal epilepsy

1.37 The prevalence of asthma increases with:

- ○ A Female sex
- ○ B Family history of eczema
- ○ C Forceps delivery
- ○ D Passive smoking during pregnancy
- ○ E Urban living

1.38 Regarding infantile spasms

- ○ A They are also known as 'salaam attacks'
- ○ B They usually start after 9 months
- ○ C They characteristically involve 'drop attacks' secondary to brief myoclonus or atonia
- ○ D Electroencephalogram (EEG) characteristically shows hypsarrhythmia in approximately 66%
- ○ E First-line treatment involves prednisolone or adrenocorticotropic hormone (ACTH)

1.39 Cerebral palsy

- ○ A is a contraindication to the pertussis vaccine
- ○ B may be secondary to hypoglycaemia in the perinatal period
- ○ C features include the lack of primitive reflexes
- ○ D may be associated with impaired hearing
- ○ E feeding difficulties arise from hypotonia

1.40 Risk factors for physical abuse include:

- ○ A Having a stepfather
- ○ B Recent parental divorce
- ○ C Birth at 31 weeks' gestation
- ○ D Being a child aged between 4 and 8 years
- ○ E Having grandparents living nearby

1.41 Regarding pica

- ○ A It is defined as 'eating of things that are not food'
- ○ B It is usually an isolated behaviour
- ○ C The 'mouthing' of objects seen at about eight months is a good example
- ○ D It is associated with iron deficiency anaemia
- ○ E Pica that does not respond to disciplinary approaches may require referral to a community paediatrician

1.42 Concerning hyperkinetic syndrome (attention deficit disorder or ADD)

- ○ A There is a boy:girl ratio of 10:1
- ○ B It may be associated with lead poisoning
- ○ C It may be associated with food additives
- ○ D It has an incidence of 5–10% in the USA
- ○ E Behavioural therapy is the mainstay of treatment

1.43 Regarding salicylate poisoning

- A It can cause respiratory alkalosis
- B It can cause metabolic acidosis
- C It can cause hypoglycaemia
- D The child may be discharged if the 4-hour serum salicylate level is 800 mg/l
- E Treatment may involve vitamin K and fresh frozen plasma (FFP)

1.44 Regarding tuberculin testing

- A It traditionally involves an injection into the extensor surface of the left forearm
- B The Heaf test should ideally be read between 48 and 72 hours
- C A positive result occurs when the area of induration is > 5 mm
- D Is negative if the Heaf grade is '1'
- E Induration > 15 mm requires further investigation and possible antituberculous chemotherapy

1.45 In sickle cell anaemia

- A approximately 10% of Afro-Caribbeans in the UK carry haemoglobin (Hb)S
- B heterozygotes show hypochromia, target cells, Howell–Jolly bodies and occasional sickle cells on their blood film
- C an antenatal diagnosis can be made
- D homozygotes are at an increased risk of biliary colic
- E painful crises develop from about 6 months of age in homozygotes

EXTENDED MATCHING QUESTIONS

1.46 Theme: Analysis of blood gases

A Compensated metabolic acidosis
B Compensated respiratory acidosis
C Metabolic acidosis
D Metabolic alkalosis
E Mixed metabolic/respiratory acidosis
F Mixed metabolic/respiratory alkalosis
G Partially compensated metabolic acidosis
H Partially compensated respiratory acidosis
I Respiratory acidosis
J Respiratory alkalosis

For each of the following cases please choose the most appropriate analysis of the blood gas results from the above list. Each item may be used once or not at all.

1 An ex 23-week gestation baby is discharged with home oxygen. His venous blood gas analysis before discharge shows: pH 7.39, $PaCO_2$ 12.1, PaO_2 6.1, HCO_3^- 42, BE (base excess) +13.

2 A 6-year-old known diabetic child presents with an intercurrent illness. His BM (blood glucose testing strip) is 25 and an arterial blood gas shows: pH 7.32, $PaCO_2$ 2.9, PaO_2 10.2, HCO_3^- 18, BE –7.

3 A 7-week-old newborn girl presents with vomiting. A capillary blood gas shows pH 7.46, $PaCO_2$ 6.4, PaO_2 5.5, HCO_3^- 38, BE +4.

questions

1.47 Theme: Vaccinations

A No live vaccines
B No vaccines at all
C Normal immunisation schedule
D Normal immunisation schedule with substitution of inactivated for live polio vaccine
E Normal schedule and conjugate pneumococcal vaccine
F Normal schedule and unconjugated pneumococcal vaccination
G Normal schedule with substitution of inactivated for live polio vaccine and no BCG
H Normal schedule with substitution of inactivated for live polio vaccine, and without MMR
I Normal schedule without MMR
J Normal schedule without MMR or BCG

For each of the following children please choose the most appropriate immunisation policy from the above list. Each item may be used once or not at all.

1 A child born in the UK with vertically acquired human immunodeficiency virus (HIV) infection.

2 A child whose sibling is undergoing treatment for acute lymphoblastic leukaemia.

3 A child who has sickle cell trait.

1.48 Theme: Infant milk formulae

A Breast milk
B Elemental formula
C 'Follow on' milk
D Goat's milk
E High-energy formula
F Hydrolysed protein formula
G Pre-term infant formula
H Term infant formula
I Soya infant formula
J Soya milk

For each of the following cases please choose the most appropriate milk from the above list. Each item may be used once or not at all.

1 A 7-month-old infant who has chronic lung disease of prematurity and is on home O_2 and is failing to thrive on term infant formula.

2 A newborn baby whose mother has hepatitis C.

3 A 2-month-old baby who suffers from gastro-oesophageal reflux, is failing to thrive and has a sibling who 'can't have dairy'.

1.49 Theme: Epilepsy

A Absence epilepsy
B Complex partial seizures (of the temporal lobe)
C Febrile convulsion
D Idiopathic generalised tonic-clonic epilepsy
E Infantile spasms
F Night terror
G Partial seizure
H Pseudoseizure
I Rigors
J Rolandic epilepsy

For each of the following cases please choose the most likely diagnosis from the above list. Each item may be used once or not at all.

1 A 8-year-old boy develops generalised tonic-clonic seizures. They occur any time during the day and can occur at night. He has centro-temporal spikes on EEG.

2 The EEG of 5-year-old child with poor concentration at school shows 3/s spike and wave discharge provoked by hyperventilation.

3 A 6-year-old child has episodes of nausea and abdominal pain, followed by repetitive chewing and jerking of the left arm for 1–2 minutes. He is confused afterwards.

1.50 Theme: Skin rashes

A Erysipelas
B Hand, foot and mouth disease
C Infectious mononucleosis
D Measles
E Molluscum contagiosum
F Pityriasis rosea
G Rubella
H Sixth disease
I Slapped cheek syndrome
J Varicella zoster

For each of the following clinical scenarios please choose the most likely diagnosis from the above list. Each item may be used once or not at all.

1 A 5-year-old boy presents with a macular rash on the trunk, some of the macules run parallel to his ribs. His mother reports that 5 days ago there was only one spot that must have spread.

2 A 4-year-old child is systemically unwell, she has erythematous cheeks that are hot and very tender to touch.

3 A 14-month-old baby girl presents with a fine pink macular rash that started on her face and spread to her trunk. Cervical and occipital lymph nodes are easily palpable.

questions

1.51 Theme: Renal diseases

A Bartter's syndrome
B Factitious illness
C Haemolytic uraemic syndrome (HUS)
D Henoch–Schönlein purpura (HSP) nephritis
E Mesangial IgA nephropathy
F Nephrotic syndrome
G Post-streptococcal glomerulonephritis
H Reflux nephropathy
I Systemic lupus erythematosus (SLE)
J Urinary tract infection

For each of the following clinical scenarios please choose the most likely diagnosis from the above list. Each item may be used once or not at all.

1 A 4-year-old child is brought to see you as his mother noticed his urine is pink. He has been complaining of headaches. His blood pressure is 130/88 mmHg. Blood tests reveal: Na^+ 130 mmol/l, K^+ 4.9 mmol/l, Urea (Ur) 12 mmol/l, Creatnine (Cr) 96 μmol/l. C_3 is reduced but C_4 is normal. Albumin is 29 g/l.

2 A 13-year-old child presents with blood in the urine. He reports having an upper respiratory tract infection (URTI) 3 days ago. His blood pressure is 120/60 mmHg. Urine analysis reveals only blood 3+, protein 2+. Renal function is normal. Complement levels are normal.

3 A 6-year-old child who has had diarrhoea for the past week is brought to A&E. Her baseline bloods reveal: Na^+ 133 mmol/l, K^+ 5.4 mmol/l, Cr 90 μmol/l, Ur 42 mmol/l, Hb 6.3 g/dl, white cell count (WCC) 2.3 × 10^9/l, platelets (plts) 95 × 10^9/l.

1.52 Theme: The unwell infant

A Cardiac failure
B Congenital toxoplasmosis
C Delayed group B streptococcal sepsis
D Delayed haemorrhagic disease of the newborn
E Duct-dependant cardiac lesion
F Galactosaemia
G Hereditary lactic acidosis
H Meningitis
I Non-accidental injury (NAI)
J Wilson's disease

For each of the following 'unwell infant' scenarios please choose the most likely diagnosis from the above list. Each item may be used once or not at all.

1 A 3-week-old baby is brought to A&E – he has recently been having problems completing his feeds and today appears short of breath. On examination he has 4-cm hepatomegaly. All blood tests are normal.

2 A 2-week-old baby boy presents to A&E, he looks unwell. He is jaundiced, peripherally shutdown and has hepato-splenomegaly. Baseline investigations show: Hb 8 g/dl, WCC 2.9×10^9/l, plts 120×10^9/l, international normalised ratio (INR) 8.6, γ-glutamyl transferase (γ-GT) 300 IU/l, BM 2.3, urine reducing sugars +ve.

3 A 6-week-old bottle-fed baby boy attends A&E with his parents. His father reports that he is always crying. On examination he is afebrile, irritable and has a bulging fontanelle. Urgent computed tomography (CT) (brain) shows multiple haemorrhages and generalised oedema.

1.53 Theme: Essential nutrients

A Calcium
B Folic acid
C Iron
D Vitamin A
E Vitamin B_6
F Vitamin B_{12}
G Vitamin C
H Vitamin D
I Vitamin E
J Zinc

For each of the cases below please choose the nutritional element most likely to be deficient from the above list. Each item may be used once or not at all.

1 A 6-year-old boy with cystic fibrosis is thought to have poor compliance with his medicines. He is failing to thrive and has mild ataxia and weakness.

2 A 4-year-old's parents are strict vegans. He is given iron supplements but is noted to be pale. His Hb is 9.2.

3 A 2-year-old child is still exclusively breast fed and has not yet started walking. He has prominent wrists and lumps round his sternum.

1.54 Theme: Respiratory conditions

A α-1 anti-trypsin
B Atopic asthma
C Cystic fibrosis
D Foreign body inhalation
E Kartagener's syndrome
F *Mycoplasma* infection
G Pertussis
H Recurrent aspiration
I Vascular ring
J Tuberculosis

For each of the following cases please choose the most likely diagnosis from the above list. Each item may be used once or not at all.

1 A 2-year-old is referred with difficulty in breathing. She is noted to be wheezy – more on the right than left. A chest X-ray reveals right-sided hyperexpansion.

2 An 18-month-old infant of a travelling family presents with an acute respiratory illness. Investigations at the time show a marked lymphocytosis. He has a persistent cough 2 months later.

3 A 3-year-old child has a recurrent nocturnal cough. He had mild eczema as an infant. He is otherwise well.

BEST OF FIVE QUESTIONS

1.55 A newborn infant is noted to be profoundly hypotonic at birth, he has a good heart rate but is in respiratory distress. Which of the following syndromes is most likely to be the cause?

- A Down's syndrome
- B Prader–Willi
- C Noonan's syndrome
- D Werdnig–Hoffman disease (spinomuscular atrophy type 1)
- E Beckwith–Wiedemann syndrome

1.56 In a child whose asthma is not controlled on a regular inhaled steroids and occasional β_2-agonist, the single next best step would be to:

- A Add long-acting β_2-agonist
- B Increase dose of inhaled steroid
- C Check inhaler technique
- D Add a leukotriene inhibitor
- E Add a short course of oral steroids

1.57 A 4-month-old infant presents with a fever, cough and reduced feeds. Her respiratory rate is 60 with mild recession, wheeze and crackles throughout. The most likely diagnosis is:

- A Croup
- B Viral-induced atopic wheeze
- C Cystic fibrosis
- D Bacterial chest infection
- E Bronchiolitis

1.58 Which one of the following statements is most correct regarding the consent for an operation on a 10-year-old child whose parents aren't married?

- ○ A Either of the parents or the child can consent to the operation
- ○ B Either of the parents but not the child can consent to the operation
- ○ C Only the mother or the child can consent to the operation
- ○ D Only the mother can consent to the operation
- ○ E Only the child can consent to the operation

1.59 Which of the following is the first sign of puberty in girls?

- ○ A Menarche
- ○ B Breast development
- ○ C Growth spurt
- ○ D Axillary hair development
- ○ E Pubic hair development

1.60 A 7-year-old boy presents with pain in his right leg. He is afebrile. On examination you note that the range of movement in his right hip is limited by pain. The most likely diagnosis is:

- ○ A Perthes' disease
- ○ B Irritable hip
- ○ C Septic arthritis
- ○ D Slipped upper femoral epiphysis (SUFE)
- ○ E Osgood–Schlatter's disease

questions

1.61 Which one of the following statements best describes clinical governance?

- ○ A Performance of audit, audit direct process change and completion of cycles
- ○ B Comprehensive risk assessment and incident reporting
- ○ C Implementation and systematic review of clinical effectiveness
- ○ D Modification of healthcare systems to optimise patient care
- ○ E Systematic training of healthcare workers to effect quality provision

1.62 A child with congenital hypothyroidism is currently on 50 μg/day of thyroxine. She is seen in clinic and has the following thyriod function tests (TFTs): free thyroxine – 20.2 (12–24) nmol/l, TSH 9.8 (1.2–4.0) mU/l. Which of the following explanations is the most likely?

- ○ A Under-treatment
- ○ B Over-treatment
- ○ C Anti-T_4 antibodies
- ○ D Poor compliance
- ○ E Wrong diagnosis

1.63 A parent suspects that her 2-year-old son has a food intolerance and wants 'tests'. He is well and growing along the appropriate centile. What is the most appropriate course of action?

- ○ A Advise her that there are no investigations that can 100% determine food intolerances
- ○ B Advise her to try to exclude the suspected food and see if this produces an improvement in his symptoms – if so then reintroduce and see if the symptoms return
- ○ C Perform skin prick testing to the suspected allergen and other common allergens
- ○ D Perform radioallergosorbent test (RAST) to the suspected allergens and other common allergens
- ○ E Perform baseline coeliac screen, stool reducing sugars, and inflammatory markers to exclude more serious pathology

1.64 A 2-month-old baby girl is brought to your surgery as her mother is concerned about a 1-cm lump situated lateral to her right eyebrow. The lump is firm and not attached to the skin. Which one of the following lumps is the most likely diagnosis?

- ○ A Enlarged lymph node
- ○ B Lipoma
- ○ C Branchial cyst
- ○ D External angular dermoid
- ○ E Neurofibroma

1.65 Which one of the following gross motor milestones would you expect a normally developing 10-month-old infant to have most recently acquired?

- A Sitting unsupported
- B Pulling to stand
- C Rolling prone to supine
- D Walking up stairs with support
- E Transferring hand to hand

1.66 Which one of the following fine motor milestones would you expect a normally developing 20-month-old infant to have most recently acquired?

- A Casting
- B Thumb/ finger grip
- C Banging two cubes together
- D Feeding self with a spoon
- E Building a tower of two cubes

1.67 A 3-year-old girl was hit by a reversing car (5 mph). She sustained a head injury and loss of consciousness for 1 minute. Subsequent to that she has vomited three times. On examination her Glasgow Coma Score (GCS) is 15/15 and there is no focal neurology. Which one of the following is the most appropriate course of action?

- A Discharge with head injury advice for the parents
- B Arrange an urgent CT scan of her brain
- C Arrange anteroposterior (AP) and lateral skull X-rays
- D Admit for 24 hours of neurological observations
- E Observe for 4 hours in A&E and then send home with head injury advice if well

1.68 Which one of the following language milestones would you expect 90% of normally developing children to have most recently developed by 1 year?

- A Turning to voice
- B Imitate speech sounds
- C Three words
- D Dada/mama (specific to person)
- E Expressive babbling

1.69 Which one of the following tests is the most appropriate to check the hearing of a 5-year-old child?

- A Auditory brainstem-evoked response
- B Distraction test
- C Oto-acoustic emissions
- D Pure tone audiometry
- E Impedance audiometry

1.70 A 3-month-old baby girl is brought to your clinic as her mother is concerned that her birthmark is still present. On examination she has a capillary haemangioma on her left thigh. Which one of the following statements is the most appropriate to tell the mother?

- A The birthmark should resolve by 5 years of age
- B The birthmark may get larger until 2 years of age then resolve by 5 years
- C The birthmark may get larger until 2 years of age then resolve by 10 years
- D The birthmark may get larger until 2 years of age and probably will have gone by 5 years but may never resolve completely
- E The birthmark may get larger until 2 years of age, and 70% resolve by 5 years and 95% by 10 years

questions

1.71 Which of the following investigations is the one that has the greatest relevance to the ophthalmic monitoring of a child with juvenile idiopathic arthritis?

- A Anti-neutrophil cytoplasmic antibodies
- B Erythrocyte sedimentation rate
- C C-reactive protein
- D Anti-nuclear antibodies (ANA)
- E Extractable nuclear antigens

1.72 Which of the following is, ideally, the most appropriate insulin regimen for a 3-year-old child newly diagnosed as an insulin-dependent diabetic?

- A Basal–bolus regimen
- B Twice daily: (30% short/70% intermediate acting) at 2/3 am 1/3 pm
- C Twice daily: (20% short/80% intermediate acting) at 1/2 am 1/2 pm
- D Once-daily long-acting insulin
- E Thrice-daily short-acting insulin

1.73 A 7-month-old baby boy from the Indian subcontinent has been in the UK for 1 month. At a routine health visit he is noted to be pale. Subsequent investigations show full blood count (FBC): Hb 9.3 g/dl, WCC 4.5 × 10^9, plts 240 × 10^9/l, mean corpuscular volume (MCV) 70 fl, ferritin 16 ng/ml, reticulocytes 1.6%, Hb electrophoresis 98% HbA. Given these results what is the most likely cause for the anaemia?

- A Physiological anaemia of infancy
- B α-Thalassaemia trait
- C Chronic helminth infection
- D Dietary iron deficiency
- E Dietary folate deficiency

1.74 A 4-year-old child presents following a viral URTI with bruising and petechiae but is afebrile and well. On examination there are petechiae on the trunk and legs, bruises on the leg, no petechiae in the mouth or lips and no other abnormal findings. His platelet count is 9×10^9, the rest of the FBC, coagulation screen and urine dipstick are normal. A diagnosis of ITP (immune-mediated thrombocytopenia purpura) is made. What is the best course of action from this point?

- ○ A Admit and observe for 48 hours with daily platelet counts
- ○ B Admit and start iv immunoglobulin
- ○ C Admit and start iv immunoglobulin followed by 1 unit of platelets
- ○ D Admit and arrange for a bone marrow aspiration with a view to starting steroids
- ○ E Discharge home but arrange for daily review and FBCs

PAPER 2

MULTIPLE CHOICE QUESTIONS

2.1 Regarding consent

- ○ A A child below 16 years of age may give consent for elective medical treatment
- ○ B If a child below 16 years of age refuses surgery it must not be carried out
- ○ C An unmarried father has both financial and intrinsic rights for his child
- ○ D If a divorced couple disagree about the need for an elective tonsillectomy in their child, the mother's opinion prevails
- ○ E If emergency surgery is needed and the parents are unavailable, consent must be obtained from a person such as a teacher who is *in loco parentis*

2.2 Regarding acne

- ○ A It affects 90% of teenagers and 25% of infants
- ○ B It is usually caused by excessive levels of testosterone
- ○ C *Propionibacterium acnes* is an anaerobic diphtheroid
- ○ D In moderate cases, treatment with erythromycin should continue for at least 6–12 months
- ○ E Roaccutane (isotretinoin – a vitamin A analogue) can be tried by the GP for severe cases resistant to all other therapy

2.3 Signs of physical abuse include:

- ◯ A Petechial rash over the child's face
- ◯ B Torn fraenum
- ◯ C Mongolian blue spot
- ◯ D Multiple bruising of various ages on the shins of a 7-year-old boy
- ◯ E Metaphyseal avulsion fractures

2.4 Regarding Turner's syndrome

- ◯ A It affects one in 2500 women
- ◯ B It has the genotype (XY); however, intrauterine development persists as female due to lack of receptors for circulating testosterone
- ◯ C It is associated with Crohn's disease
- ◯ D Features apparent at birth include a webbed neck, low posterior hairline and widely spaced nipples
- ◯ E Somatotrophin (human growth hormone) is a useful treatment for short stature once the epiphyses have fused

2.5 Regarding *Molluscum contagiosum*

- ◯ A It is a pox RNA virus infection
- ◯ B It typically presents with small pearly umbilicated lesions anywhere on the body
- ◯ C It has low infectivity
- ◯ D Lesions generally take 6–9 months to resolve
- ◯ E The treatment of choice is removal by piercing the lesion with a sharpened orange stick dipped in phenol or liquid nitrogen

2.6 Regarding nappy rash

- A It typically involves the flexures when due to irritant dermatitis
- B A red rash with satellite lesions and shallow ulcers is typical of candidiasis
- C It frequently becomes secondarily infected with *Staphylococcus aureus*
- D Topical Dermovate cream (clobetasol propionate) is the treatment of choice for the scaly intertriginous nappy rash
- E Nappy rash due to seborrhoeic dermatitis may be associated with cradle cap

2.7 With regard to factitious or induced illness

- A It has a mortality of 2–10%
- B Confrontation with evidence should be avoided
- C It never involves the father
- D The child may show evidence of failure to thrive
- E Generally occurs in pre-school children

2.8 Regarding club foot

- A It is more common in boys
- B The feet are held in equinovalgus
- C It may be associated with spina bifida
- D It will need surgical repair
- E Treatment should be commenced at the age of 3 months

2.9 Regarding cleft lip

- A It has an equal incidence among boys and girls
- B It is increasing in incidence
- C It affects approximately 1 in 750 live births
- D It is associated with cleft palate in less than 20% of cases
- E The risk to a child whose sibling has a cleft lip is 5%

2.10 With regard to tonsillectomy

- A It is indicated in children having two attacks of tonsillitis a year
- B Complications include development of a quinsy
- C It should be performed if parents request a prophylactic procedure
- D Complications include complete dysphagia
- E Post-operative secondary haemorrhage is treated with antibiotics

2.11 Regarding Wilms' nephroblastoma

- A It commonly presents before 5 years of age
- B It is frequently bilateral
- C It often presents with haematuria
- D Diagnosis should be confirmed by renal biopsy
- E It is the most common intra-abdominal tumour of childhood

2.12 Regarding undescended testis

- A It is present in 15–30% of term male infants
- B When present it is usually bilateral
- C It is most commonly found at the superficial inguinal pouch
- D Orchidopexy should be performed before 4 years of age
- E It has an increased incidence of torsion

2.13 Known side-effects of sodium valproate include:

- A Pancreatitis
- B Stevens–Johnson syndrome
- C Hyperactivity, commonly
- D Increased appetite and obesity
- E Epigastric pain and nausea

2.14 An acute asthma attack may be triggered by:

- ○ A Exercise
- ○ B Gastro-oesophageal reflux
- ○ C Climatic change
- ○ D Rhinovirus infection
- ○ E Emotion

2.15 With regard to Bacillus Calmette-Guérin (BCG)

- ○ A High-risk infants should have a positive Heaf test before vaccination proceeds
- ○ B It is safe in asymptomatic HIV-positive patients
- ○ C It may be given at the same time as other live vaccines
- ○ D It should be given after a positive tuberculin test
- ○ E Offers some protection against leprosy

2.16 Congenital rubella is characteristically associated with:

- ○ A Deafness with maternal infection at 10–16 weeks' gestation
- ○ B Retinopathy
- ○ C Hydrocephalus
- ○ D Polycythaemia
- ○ E Neonatal conjugated hyperbilirubinaemia

2.17 Which of these definitions is correct?

- A The 'incidence' of influenza is much lower than its 'prevalence'
- B The 'perinatal mortality' is the number of stillbirths and deaths within the first week of life per 1000 total births
- C 'Stillbirth rate' is the number of stillbirths per 1000 total births
- D 'Neonatal mortality rate' (NMR) is the number of deaths up to 1 month of age per 1000 total births
- E 'Infant mortality rate' (IMR) is the number of deaths under 1 year

2.18 With regard to Apgar scores

- A A heart rate of < 100 bpm scores 1
- B Approximately 45% of all babies whose Apgar score is < 4 at 5 minutes will die
- C They are recorded at 0, 1 and 5 minutes
- D They are not used in intubated babies
- E A blue baby scores 0

2.19 Features linked to depression in a child of 10 years may include:

- A Diabetes mellitus
- B Epilepsy
- C Primary enuresis
- D Abdominal pain
- E Recent vandalism

2.20 Regarding developmental dysplasia of the hip

○ A It is more common in boys
○ B It occurs in 5–20 per 1000 live births
○ C It affects the right hip more than the left
○ D The diagnosis should be confirmed by USS
○ E It is associated with a breech presentation

2.21 Features of cystic fibrosis include:

○ A Rectal prolapse
○ B Prolonged neonatal jaundice
○ C Digital clubbing
○ D Failure to thrive
○ E *Pseudomonas* chest infection

2.22 Roseola infantum

○ A presents with a rash on the first day
○ B has an incubation period of approximately 5–15 days
○ C is commonly due to herpes virus type 6
○ D is also known as 'fifth disease'
○ E is associated with pneumonia

2.23 Causes of tall stature include:

○ A Constitutional
○ B Homocystinuria
○ C Hyperthyroidism
○ D Pseudohypoparathyroidism
○ E Cushing's syndrome

2.24 Regarding the treatment of asthma

- A Aminophylline cannot be given if the child is already on regular oral theophylline
- B Cromoglycate is a useful agent in the treatment of acute asthma
- C Inhalers deliver less than 5% of the drug to the lungs
- D The incidence of oral candidiasis can be reduced if steroids are inhaled via a spacer device
- E Regular inhaled low-dose steroids do not result in growth retardation

2.25 Examples of primary prevention include:

- A Cycling helmets
- B Stair gates
- C Teaching children road safety from a young age
- D Smoke alarms
- E Child-proof catches on cupboards

2.26 The Dubowitz system for assessment of gestational age include the following external criteria:

- A Nipple formation
- B Ear firmness
- C Nail development
- D Presence of eyelashes
- E Breast size

2.27 Infants born to poorly controlled diabetic mothers may have:

- A Erb's palsy
- B Sacral agenesis
- C Hypomagnesaemia
- D Hypercalcaemia
- E Anaemia

2.28 Regarding the management of UTIs

- ○ A Amoxicillin is the first-line treatment in children
- ○ B Prophylactic antibiotics are given four times daily for 1 month
- ○ C It includes avoiding constipation
- ○ D Asymptomatic bacteriuria should always be treated with appropriate antibiotics
- ○ E It may involve surgery

2.29 Cerebral palsy

- ○ A is a progressive condition
- ○ B has a prevalence of 2.5 in 1000
- ○ C is associated with a mental handicap in 70–80% of cases
- ○ D is due to perinatal hypoxic-ischaemic injury in the majority of cases
- ○ E may present with clumsiness

2.30 The stepwise treatment of asthma involves

- ○ A Step 2: the regular use of low-dose inhaled steroids and bronchodilators as required
- ○ B Starting at 'step 1' and gradually stepping up treatment until an appropriate level is reached
- ○ C Step 4: the regular use of high-dose systemic steroids
- ○ D 'Stepping down' if control has been good for over 3 months
- ○ E Step 5: the addition of slow release xanthine, ± nebulised β-agonist, ± alternate day prednisolone, ± ipratropium or β-agonist subcutaneous infusion

2.31 Regarding the epidemiology of asthma

- A Asthma causes approximately 50 deaths per year in the UK
- B The majority of deaths occur amongst 0- to 4-year-olds
- C Asthma affects 2–5% of all children in the UK
- D The prevalence has gradually been decreasing over the past 20 years
- E The mortality rate has gradually been decreasing over the past 10 years

2.32 Concerning cystic fibrosis

- A The gene for cystic fibrosis is located on the long arm of chromosome 7
- B It may be diagnosed antenatally by chorionic villous biopsy
- C The risk of two carriers having an affected child is 1 in 2
- D It has a gene carrier rate of 1 in 40 in the Caucasian population
- E Approximately 75–80% of cystic fibrosis gene mutations in the UK are due to a deletion at delta F508

2.33 With respect to generalised 'absences'

- A They are more common in girls
- B They are associated with mental disability
- C 30% go on to develop generalised tonic-clonic epilepsy
- D The EEG shows unilateral spike waves over the Rolandic area
- E First-line treatment is carbamazepine

2.34 Chronic constipation

- A often presents with diarrhoea
- B is normal in breast-fed babies
- C is frequently diet related
- D is associated with Down's syndrome
- E is defined as the infrequent passage of stools

2.35 Regarding case conferences for child abuse

- ○ A The Butler–Schloss report recommends that parents must always be invited to attend the case conference
- ○ B They should ideally be held during the Emergency Protection Order (EPO)
- ○ C The GP should be invited to attend
- ○ D They have only the capacity to decide whether the child should be placed on the Child Protection Register
- ○ E They must be attended by a senior officer from the social services

2.36 Reye's syndrome

- ○ A is acute encephalopathy with fatty degeneration of the liver, kidneys and pancreas
- ○ B is associated with ibuprofen exposure in young children
- ○ C usually presents before the age of 2 years
- ○ D is commonly complicated by hypoglycaemia
- ○ E alanine aminotransferase (ALT), aspartate aminotransferase (AST) and bilirubin are usually elevated

2.37 Regarding Fallot's tetralogy

- ○ A It typically has a left-to-right shunt
- ○ B It typically has a pansystolic murmur
- ○ C Cyanotic spells may be prevented by treatment with β-blockers
- ○ D It has the characteristic chest X-ray appearance of an 'egg lying on its side'
- ○ E Fallot's tetralogy and the transposition of the great arteries (TGA) are the two leading causes of cyanotic congenital heart disease

2.38 Features of a headache that would support the diagnosis of a simple migraine includes:

- A being preceded by transient visual field defects and micropsia
- B Papilloedema
- C Strabismus
- D Diplopia
- E Nystagmus

2.39 Regarding Down's syndrome

- A It is associated with an increased incidence of duodenal atresia
- B It is the single most common cause of severe learning difficulty
- C It is associated with hypothyroidism
- D Trisomy 21 has a recurrence risk of 10%
- E It is associated with general hypertonia

2.40 With reagrd to haemophilia

- A Haemophilia B is an autosomal recessive disorder
- B Children with haemophilia A must never be given aspirin
- C The prothrombin time is normal in both haemophilia A and B
- D Regular dental care is essential
- E It is associated with progressive joint destruction

2.41 In chronic diarrhoea

- ○ A In the UK, cows' milk protein intolerance is the most common cause of chronic diarrhoea in infants under 1 year
- ○ B Recognisable food in the stool suggests toddler diarrhoea
- ○ C Flat mucosa devoid of villa on a jejunal biopsy is diagnostic of coeliac disease
- ○ D Coeliac disease most commonly presents between 6 and 9 months of age
- ○ E Ulcerative colitis is inherited in an autosomal recessive manner

2.42 Regarding appendicitis

- ○ A It is rare in the under-fives (< 2%)
- ○ B In the under-fives, nearly 90% of cases present with perforation
- ○ C Abdominal pain usually presents in the right iliac fossa
- ○ D Its differential diagnosis includes mesenteric adenitis, UTI and diabetic ketoacidosis
- ○ E Assessing the child's ability to 'hop' helps exclude the diagnosis

2.43 The role of the health visitor includes:

- ○ A Supervising the running of immunisation clinics
- ○ B Reviewing every child under 5 years who has attended the A&E Department
- ○ C Child health surveillance in all children under 10 years of age
- ○ D Taking over postnatal care from the midwife at 3 weeks of age
- ○ E Responsibility for supervision of children in care

questions

2.44 Regarding anorexia nervosa

- A It affects 1 in 250 girls between the ages of 15 and 18 years
- B Primary amenorrhoea may be present
- C It is associated with hyperkalaemia
- D It has a mortality rate of 1%
- E It is characterised by having a disturbed perception of body image

2.45 Ophthalmology

- A Ophthalmia neonatorum is most commonly caused by *Neisseria gonorrhoeae*
- B Stevens–Johnson syndrome is associated with iritis
- C Orbital cellulitis is commonly secondary to adjacent sinusitis
- D Glaucoma may be associated with aniridia
- E Intrauterine toxoplasmosis infection results in an increased incidence of cataracts

EXTENDED MATCHING QUESTIONS

2.46 Theme: Choice of investigations

A Blood cultures
B Bone marrow aspiration cytology
C Clotting screen
D C-reactive protein
E Erythrocyte sedimentation rate
F FBC
G G-6-PD assay
H Haemoglobin electrophoresis
I Monospot
J Peripheral blood film

For each of the following cases please choose the investigation most likely to give a definitive diagnosis from the above list. Each item may be used once or not at all.

1 A 6-month-old Afro-Caribbean infant presents with dactylitis.

2 A 7-year-old girl, who had an URTI 1 week ago, bruises easily and has developed petechiae.

3 A 14-year-old boy who presents with a sore throat and palatal petechiae.

2.47 Theme: Decisions about life-saving treatment

A The brain-dead child
B The 'no chance' situation
C The 'no purpose' situation
D The persistent vegetative state
E The 'unbearable' situation

For each of the following cases please choose the most appropriate criterion under which life-saving treatment could be withdrawn (as identified by the Royal College of Paediatrics and Child Health (RCPCH)) from the above list. Each item may be used once or not at all.

1 A 4-year-old girl who, despite maximal intensive care, is deteriorating due to meningococcal septicaemia.

2 A 5-year-old boy who has relapsed for the third time with acute myeloblastic leukaemia and doesn't wish for further chemotherapy.

3 A 1-year-old, who having sustained such severe head injuries in a road traffic accident that he is expected to be profoundly brain damaged, develops a pneumonia whilst in the paediatric intensive care unit (PICU).

2.48 Theme: Heart defects

A Aortic stenosis
B ASD
C Coarctation of the aorta
D Ebstein's anomaly
E Innocent (flow) murmur
F PDA
G Pulmonary stenosis
H Tetralogy of Fallot
I Transposition of the great arteries
J Ventricular septal defect

For each of the following sets of clinical findings please choose the most likely diagnosis from the above list. Each item may be used once or not at all.

1 A 3-year-old child presents to his GP with a febrile illness and is noted to have a soft ejection systolic murmur at the left sternal edge (LSE) only.

2 A 12-hour-old newborn baby, at her discharge check, is noted to have a pansystolic murmur heard all over the praecordium. The femoral pulses are very easily palpable.

3 A baby girl is seen for the 8-week check and is noted to have an ejection systolic murmur best heard in the pulmonary area. The second heart sound does not vary with respiration. There is 1-cm hepatomegaly.

2.49 Theme: Common infections

A Adenovirus
B β-Haemolytic streptococcus
C Coxsackie virus A16
D Epstein–Barr virus (EBV)
E Human herpesvirus 6
F *Mycoplasma pneumoniae*
G Parvovirus B19
H Poxvirus
I Rhinovirus
J Varicella zoster virus

For each of the following scenarios please choose the most likely underlying causative organism from the above list. Each item may be used once or not at all.

1 A 12-year-old boy has a painful erythematous throat for which he is prescribed a broad-spectrum antibiotic. He re-presents the following day with a florid macular-papular rash all over his trunk.

2 A 3-year-old is at nursery and her mother notices that she is unwell, refusing foods and has some vesicles on her palms and toes.

3 A 7-year-old boy presents with feeling unwell and has a macular rash all over his body. There are some 'target lesions' visible.

2.50 Theme: Statistics and research methods

A Incidence
B Lag time
C Lead time
D Length bias
E Likelihood ratio
F Number needed to treat
G Paired cohort
H Prevalence
I Sensitivity
J Specificity

For each of the following definitions please choose the word that applies to it from the above list. Each item may be used once or not at all.

1 Interval between identification of a condition by screening and the development of symptoms.

2 Odds of a positive test result in an affected individual compared with that of a positive result in an unaffected individual.

3 Proportion of people unaffected by a condition correctly identified by a designated test.

questions

2.51 Theme: Immediate interventions

A Adenosine 50 μg/kg iv
B Amiodarone 5 mg/kg iv
C Asynchronous DC shock – 0.5 J/kg
D Asynchronous DC shock – 2 J/kg
E Asynchronous DC shock – 4 J/kg
F Atropine 20 μg/kg iv
G Lignocaine 1 mg/kg iv
H Sodium bicarbonate 4.2% 4 ml/kg iv
I Synchronous DC shock – 0.5 J/kg
J Vagal manoeuvres

For the cases below please choose the most appropriate immediate intervention (Airway and Breathing can be assumed to be already managed) from the above list. Each item may be used once or not at all.

1 A 3-year-old has the following trace (SVT). Her capillary refill time (CRT) is 4 s, and her O_2 saturations are 92% in 5-l O_2 by mask.

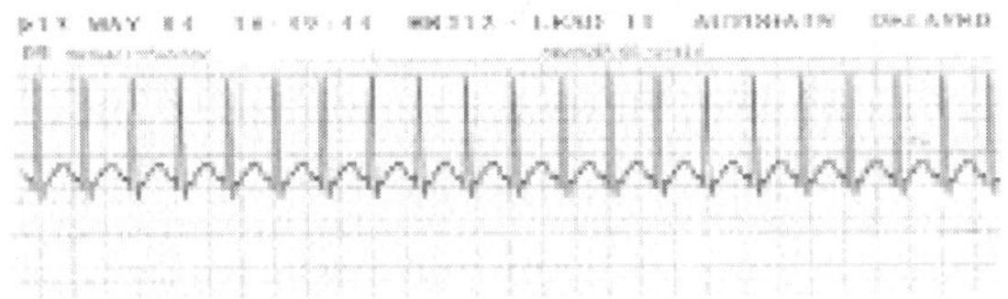

2 A 15-year-old girl with a history of deliberate self-harm presents acutely unwell. ECG monitoring shows the following trace – (VT). Her pulse is weak but present, CRT is 5 s, *S*aO_2 90% in 10-l O_2 by mask.

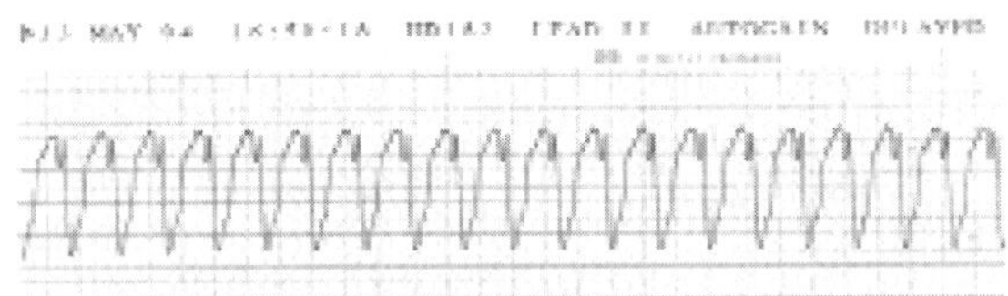

3 A 2-year-old child comes in found unresponsive by her parents. She is being ventilated by bag-valve-mask by the paramedics. She is pulseless and has this rhythm on the monitor (VF).

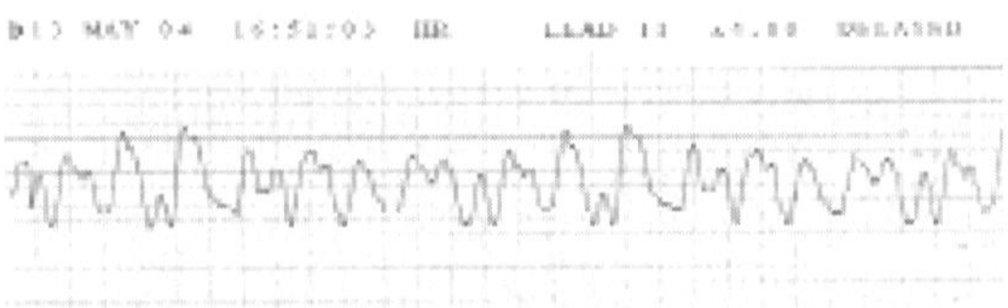

2.52 Theme: Neoplasms

A Acute myeloblastic leukaemia
B ALL
C Atrial myxoma
D Ewing's sarcoma
E Medulloblastoma
F Neuroblastoma
G Non-Hodgkin's lymphoma
H Osteosarcoma
I Rhabdomyosarcoma
J Wilms' tumour

For each of the following cases please choose the single most likely diagnosis from the above list. Each item may be used once or not at all.

1 A 2-year-old presents with a 1-month history of lethargy, not being himself and bruising easily. He has hepatosplenomegaly and an FBC reveals: Hb 9.2 g/dl, WCC 2.3×10^9/l, plts 50×10^9/l.

2 A 3-year-old boy has a large left flank mass and a trace of blood in the urine.

3 A 9-year-old boy presents with lethargy, shortness of breath and night sweats. On examination splenomegaly can be felt. There are no blast cells present on the blood film.

2.53 Theme: Gastro-intestinal disorders

A Abetalipoproteinaemia
B Coeliac disease
C Constipation with overflow
D Crohn's disease
E Giardiasis
F Ileal tuberculosis
G Lactose intolerance
H Toddler's diarrhoea
I Ulcerative colitis
J Viral gastro-enteritis

For each of the following cases please choose the most likely cause of the diarrhoea from the above list. Each item may be used once or not at all.

1 A 9-year-old boy presents with a 2-month history of weight loss, abdominal pain and intermittent diarrhoea. There is no blood in the stool. He has a mildly tender abdomen and some perianal skin tags. Investigations reveal: CRP 45 mg/dl, ESR 50 mm first hour.

2 A 3-year-old girl has a 2-month history of loose stools. Her parents are very concerned. The stools often contain 'undigested food'. She is otherwise well and thriving.

3 An 8-month-old infant has had watery diarrhoea for 4 days. There has been no recent travel. Her 2-year-old sibling has recently had a similar illness, though less severe. She is drinking her normal formula milk well and is not dehydrated.

2.54 Theme: Endocrine disorders

A Chronic corticosteroid therapy
B Cystic fibrosis
C Constitutional delay in growth and puberty
D Growth hormone deficiency
E Hypochondroplasia
F Hypothyroidism
G Psychosocial deprivation
H Rickets
I Small genetic height potential
J Turner's syndrome

For each of the following cases of poor growth please choose the most likely cause from the above list. Each item may be used once or not at all.

1 A 7-year-old girl comes to outpatients with her parents, who are concerned that she is too short. She has previously been fit and well. Her height and weight are both on the 2nd centile. Parental heights are on the 2nd (mother) and 10th (father) centiles.

2 A 13-year-old boy is the shortest in his class. He has no pubic or axillary hair and his testicular volume is 8 ml. His bone age is delayed.

3 A 9-year-old girl has previously had a bone marrow transplant (matched sibling donor) for ALL. She presents as her growth is not keeping up with her peers. She is falling behind academically. She is gaining weight and has constipation.

BEST OF FIVE QUESTIONS

2.55 Which one of the following statements best describes the circumstances in which a parent would be legally permitted to smack their child?

- A Anywhere on the body, but not on the face
- B Anywhere on the body, but only after consideration (not in the heat of the moment)
- C Anywhere on the body, as long as only the hand is used and no mark is left
- D Anywhere on the body, except the face, but only in the home and not in public
- E Anywhere on the body, as long as any implement used does not leave a mark

2.56 Which of the following is the best first-line step in management of a 5-year-old child who develops constipation after a viral illness?

- A Dietary advice
- B Seven-day trial of lactulose (10 ml bd)
- C One glycerin suppository
- D Two stat phosphate enemas
- E Admission for administration of Klean prep

2.57 A baby boy is noted to have hypospadias at the post-natal check. The meatus is situated ventrally, and a chordee is noted. The most important piece of advice to give to the parents is:

- A His adult sexual function should be normal
- B You must be careful when washing his penis
- C He must not be circumcised
- D He may require surgery in later childhood
- E Treat your baby as normal

2.58 A 15-year-old girl presents with a 2-month history of abdominal pain. She has had no fever and no other symptoms. Examination reveals 3-cm hepatomegaly and splenomegaly. The single most useful investigation would be:

- A C-reactive protein
- B Blood film
- C Abdominal USS
- D Paul Bunnell test
- E Liver function tests (LFTs) + amylase

2.59 A child who has a 2-day history of fever has a bright red, infected left tympanic membrane. The child is eating and drinking well. What would be the most appropriate course of action?

- A Referral to ENT surgeons as an emergency
- B Referral to ENT surgeons as an outpatient
- C 5-day course of oral penicillin V
- D Advice to parents that this is a self-limiting condition and is best left alone
- E Regular antipyretics and analgesics with review in 48 hours

2.60 Which of the following is the most important pathology to exclude on a cranial USS performed on day 1 of the life of a 25-week-gestation premature baby?

- A Hydrocephalus
- B Gyral pattern
- C Periventricular leukomalacia
- D Intraventricular haemorrhage
- E Cerebral atrophy

2.61 What is the most important investigation to perform in a 3-week-old newborn baby boy who is feeding well and thriving, but is referred with jaundice?

- A Direct and indirect bilirubin
- B TFTs
- C LFTs
- D Urine organic acids
- E Coombs' test

2.62 An 8-month-old infant presents to A&E with a 3-day history of frequent watery diarrhoea and vomiting. On examination she is 5% dehydrated. She is refusing to drink in the emergency department. Which one of the following is the most appropriate course of action?

- A Admit for intravenous rehydration (maintenance and 5% deficit)
- B Observe for 4 hours in the emergency department – if she tolerates oral fluids then discharge her, if not admit for iv rehydration
- C Admit for enteral rehydration via a nasogastric tube
- D Admit for iv rehydration (maintenance) + oral fluids as tolerated
- E Short course of oral cephalexin

2.63 In a mother who is hepatitis B surface antibody (sAb) +ve, and core antigen (eAg) +ve, which of the following combinations is the most appropriate for her newborn baby?

- A Hepatitis B vaccine
- B Hepatitis B immunoglobulin
- C Hepatitis B vaccine and hepatitis B immunoglobulin
- D Hepatitis B vaccine and iv pooled immunoglobulin
- E Hepatitis B and hepatitis C vaccines combined

2.64 Which one of the following social milestones would you expect a normally developing 15-month-old infant to have most recently acquired?

- A Brush teeth with help
- B Play ball with examiner
- C Wave bye-bye
- D Put on T-shirt with no help
- E Play 'pat-a-cake'

2.65 In primary nocturnal enuresis in a 5-year-old, which of the following is the most appropriate initial management strategy?

- A Family counselling
- B Star chart
- C Verbal chastisement
- D Short trial of imipramine
- E Short trial of desmopressin

2.66 Which one of the following gross motor milestones would you expect 90% of normally developing children to have most recently developed by 4 years?

- A Able to run steadily
- B Walk backwards
- C Hop on one leg
- D Walk up stairs unaided
- E Throw ball over-hand

questions

2.67 A 4-year-old girl is suffering physical abuse at home. Which one of the following interventions would be most appropriate to apply if her welfare is thought to be immediate danger?

- A Police protection order (PPO)
- B Emergency protection order
- C Court wardship
- D Section 47 meeting
- E Temporary foster placement

2.68 A 4-year-old girl suffers a femoral fracture in a road traffic accident. She also has a contusion on her right forehead. She is screaming with the pain from her leg. Which one of the following would be the most effective and safest forms of analgesia?

- A Per rectum (PR) diclofenac and oral codeine
- B Splinting of the fractured limb
- C Paracetamol, ibuprofen and codeine per os (po)
- D Morphine iv
- E Femoral nerve block

2.69 Which of the following diagnoses is the most likely in a 3-year-old boy who has epilepsy and on examination has numerous depigmented macules and two café-au-lait spots.

- A Tuberous sclerosis
- B Neurofibromatosis 1
- C Ataxia telangiectasia
- D Incontinentia pigmenti
- E Sturge–Weber syndrome

2.70 A 2-year-old Caucasian boy is diagnosed with nephrotic syndrome. Which one of the following is the most likely underlying pathology?

- ◯ A Minimal change disease
- ◯ B Mesangial proliferative disease
- ◯ C Focal segmental glomerular sclerosis
- ◯ D 'Finnish' type microcystic disease
- ◯ E Cystinosis

2.71 A 4-year-old child presents with a coryzal symptoms, cough, fever and abdominal pain. There is no dysuria and urine dipstick is unremarkable. On examination the pain is in the left upper quadrant but is not severe. Which is the most likely cause?

- ◯ A Urinary tract infection
- ◯ B Appendicitis
- ◯ C Pyelonephritis
- ◯ D Left basal chest infection
- ◯ E Mesenteric adenitis

2.72 A 6-week-old baby is referred for back arching and crying. He posits after feeds, especially when he lies on his back. He is thriving. You suspect gastro-oesophageal reflux (GOR). What is the most appropriate course of action?

- ◯ A Barium swallow
- ◯ B Trial of Gaviscon
- ◯ C Trial of domperidone and ranitidine
- ◯ D Reassure the parents
- ◯ E pH study

questions

2.73 A 15-year-old girl is referred following a deliberate paracetamol overdose. She reports having taken five pills 45 minutes ago. What is the most appropriate course of action?

- ○ A Administer activated charcoal and take paracetamol levels at 4 hours
- ○ B Administer activated charcoal and start iv *N*-acetylcysteine; then take paracetamol levels at 4 hours
- ○ C Start iv *N*-acetylcysteine, and take levels at 4 hours
- ○ D Wait and take blood at 4 hours for paracetamol levels
- ○ E Discharge her as it is not a harmful dose.

2.74 The 15-year-old girl in Q 2.73 has paracetamol levels well below the treatment line at 4 hours. She says she only took the pills as a 'cry for help' and regrets doing it. What is the most appropriate course of action?

- ○ A Discharge her with an urgent child psychiatry outpatient appointment
- ○ B Discharge her and contact the school educational psychologist
- ○ C Admit her for formal assessment by a child psychiatrist
- ○ D Admit her for observation overnight and discharge her if well the next day with a child psychiatry outpatient appointment
- ○ E Discharge her for GP follow-up

PAPER 3

MULTIPLE CHOICE QUESTIONS

3.1 Concerning secretory otitis media (glue ear)

- A It can cause sensorineural hearing loss
- B It may present as a behavioural problem
- C The primary role of the grommet is to drain the middle ear effusion
- D Most grommets require surgical removal
- E The majority of affected children will have normal hearing by 8 years of age

3.2 In *Haemophilus influenzae* type b (Hib) disease:

- A 60% of invasive Hib disease presents as meningitis
- B The mortality of Hib meningitis is approximately 20%
- C Hib infection is rare before 2 years of age
- D Hib vaccination is contraindicated in HIV-positive individuals
- E All infants in the absence of genuine contraindications should be vaccinated at 2, 3 and 4 months of age

3.3 'Health of the Nation' targets that are relevant to the health of children and adolescents include:

- A Smoking, alcohol consumption and illegal substance abuse
- B Healthy diets and prevention of obesity
- C Suicide and deliberate self-harm
- D Teenage pregnancy and sexually transmitted diseases
- E Accident prevention

3.4 Regarding growth charts

- A Infants aged 0–1 year should have at least three recordings of height and weight
- B All children below the second centile for height should be reviewed by the GP
- C All children below the first centile for height should be referred for a specialist opinion
- D Normal growth velocity of children over 2 years of age is 10 cm/year
- E Children with a growth velocity less than the 25th or greater than the 75th centile should be referred for a specialist opinion

3.5 Signs of child abuse include:

- A 'Frozen watchfulness'
- B Acute hyphaema
- C A single green/yellow bruise over the forehead of a toddler
- D A mid-clavicular fracture in a 10-day-old newborn
- E Scalds over both buttocks

3.6 With regard to dermatophyte (ringworm) infections in children

- ○ A Tinea pedis is rare in children under 5 years
- ○ B *Trichophyton* often causes tinea capitis
- ○ C Tinea corporis typically presents with hair loss, circular patches of alopecia with scaling skin and broken hairs
- ○ D These are caused by superficial filamentous (hyphae) fungal infections of skin which fluoresce under Wood's light
- ○ E Large infected areas may require a 2-week course of oral griseofulvin

3.7 Risk factors for developmental dysplasia of the hip (DDH) include:

- ○ A Male sex
- ○ B Oligohydramnios
- ○ C Sister had DDH
- ○ D Forceps delivery
- ○ E Maternal drug abuse

3.8 Signs of severe acute asthma include:

- ○ A Normal $PaCO_2$ on arterial blood gas analysis
- ○ B Agitation
- ○ C Use of accessory muscles
- ○ D Presence of pectus carinatum
- ○ E Pulsus paradoxus of 10–20 mmHg

3.9 Regarding acute epiglottitis

- A It commonly occurs in infants less than 1 year of age
- B The incidence has significantly decreased since the introduction of the Hib vaccine
- C It is associated with septicaemia
- D The child characteristically holds their head in hyperflexion
- E It should be confirmed by a lateral neck X-ray

3.10 Known side-effects of phenytoin include:

- A Megaloblastic anaemia
- B Lymphoma
- C Dyskinesia (including choreoathetosis)
- D SLE
- E Gum hypertrophy

3.11 With regard to tics

- A They are defined as stereotypic, repetitive, voluntary movements
- B Simple developmental tics affect 15% of primary school children
- C They are generally not of pathological significance and are usually outgrown by 4 years
- D They may be manifestations of tension or emotional disorder when they commonly persist beyond adolescence
- E They may be familial

3.12 Regarding childhood asthma

- ○ A Dehydration is common in asthma, so iv fluids should be increased to one-third above normal maintenance in severe cases
- ○ B A chest X-ray on admission should be taken in all children presenting with an acute exacerbation
- ○ C PEFR should be measured in children older than 5 years
- ○ D In the UK the most common reason for a child to be admitted to hospital is for an acute exacerbation of asthma
- ○ E IV steroids are first-line treatment in all cases of acute exacerbation of asthma

3.13 The MMR vaccine

- ○ A is contraindicated in patients allergic to neomycin
- ○ B should not be given within 3 weeks of another live vaccine (except OPV (Sabin))
- ○ C is safe in pregnancy
- ○ D commonly results in a rash with or without fever from day 5–10 lasting approximately 2 days
- ○ E is contraindicated in patients who have received an injection of immunoglobulin within 3 months

3.14 Maternal risk factors for increased perinatal mortality and morbidity include:

- ○ A Age between 16 and 35 years
- ○ B Short stature
- ○ C A birth interval of 18–36 months
- ○ D A twin pregnancy
- ○ E A previous ectopic pregnancy

3.15 Plagiocephaly

- A is often associated with babies who are consistently put into the cot on the same side
- B may present with torticollis at 6 months to 3 years
- C is associated with craniosynostosis
- D has an increased incidence of epilepsy
- E generally spontaneously improves with time

3.16 Known side-effects of carbamazepine include:

- A Aplastic anaemia
- B Rickets
- C Ataxia
- D Transient hair loss
- E Rash

3.17 Known side-effects of clonazepam include:

- A Salivary and bronchial hypersecretion
- B Nystagmus
- C Somnolence and hypotonia
- D Reversible leukopenia
- E Acne

3.18 Cystic fibrosis

- A affects approximately 1 in 2000 live births in the UK
- B has an X-linked inheritance
- C may present with meconium ileus
- D is associated with delayed puberty
- E is associated with nasal polyposis

3.19 Causes of haematuria include:

- ◯ A Exercise
- ◯ B Idiopathic
- ◯ C Allergy
- ◯ D Meatal stenosis
- ◯ E Malaria

3.20 Examples of secondary prevention include:

- ◯ A Seat belts
- ◯ B Blister packs for prescription drugs
- ◯ C Teaching parents first aid skills
- ◯ D Fire extinguishers kept in the house
- ◯ E Speed limits

3.21 Congenital rubella syndrome includes:

- ◯ A Deafness
- ◯ B Microphthalmia
- ◯ C Cardiac defects
- ◯ D Cerebral palsy
- ◯ E Saddle nose

3.22 Regarding congenital heart disease (CHD)

- ◯ A Down's syndrome is associated with an increased incidence of ventricular septal defect (VSD) and atrial septal defect (ASD)
- ◯ B It has an incidence of approximately 8 per 10, 000 live births
- ◯ C An indometacin infusion can be used to keep the ductus arteriosus patent until corrective surgery can be carried out.
- ◯ D VSD is the most common congenital heart defect
- ◯ E The incidence of cyanotic CHD is approximately three times that of acyanotic lesions

questions

3.23 Regarding foster care

- A Short-term fostering is usually up to 18 months
- B Long-term fostering is preferred for younger children
- C It is more likely to be successful if there are children of a similar age in the placement family
- D There is usually a limit of three foster children per family
- E Children in long-term foster care require a 6-monthly medical examination

3.24 In the treatment of asthma

- A Oral salbutamol syrup is useful in the treatment of infants and toddlers
- B A plastic coffee cup may be used as a spacer device
- C Inhaled drugs cannot be effectively delivered to children under 2 years of age
- D A 3-year-old can use dry powder inhalers
- E A spacer device is unsuitable in children over 10 years

3.25 Risk factors for sudden infant death syndrome (SIDS) include:

- A Female sex
- B Twins
- C Bottle feeding
- D Previous history of a sibling dying from SIDS
- E Supine sleeping position

3.26 Common features of cystic fibrosis include:

- A Anorexia
- B Steatorrhoea
- C A positive sweat test, where the concentration of sweat sodium is > 70 mmol/l
- D An increased incidence in the Chinese
- E Male impotence

3.27 Regarding vesico-ureteric reflux (VUR)

- ◯ A It should be routinely screened for in all children under 5 years
- ◯ B 10% of children with VUR will develop renal scarring
- ◯ C Grade II VUR involves urine refluxing into the kidney on micturition only
- ◯ D If severe it may require an endoscopic submucosal Teflon injection
- ◯ E It requires monitoring with serial USS

3.28 Regarding spastic hemiplegia

- ◯ A The legs are more severely affected than the arms
- ◯ B It may result from an infarct of the cortex or internal capsule
- ◯ C Almost all affected children walk by school age
- ◯ D One leg may be shorter than the other
- ◯ E It characteristically results in learning difficulties

3.29 Signs of sexual abuse in children include:

- ◯ A HIV infection
- ◯ B Clitoromegaly
- ◯ C Sexualised behaviour inappropriate for age
- ◯ D Anal fissures
- ◯ E Anal skin tags

3.30 Regarding acute renal failure (ARF)

- ◯ A Gentamicin is a cause of prerenal failure
- ◯ B It may be caused by haemolytic uraemic syndrome
- ◯ C It may be complicated by convulsions or tetany
- ◯ D Management should include a high-protein diet
- ◯ E An indication for dialysis is a plasma urea > 54 mmol/l

3.31 Signs of severe acute asthma include:

- ○ A Presence of a loud wheeze
- ○ B Being too breathless to eat
- ○ C Heart rate between 100 and 140 beats/min
- ○ D PEFR < 50% of predicted
- ○ E Respiratory rate > 50 breaths/min

3.32 Regarding infantile colic

- ○ A It characteristically presents with paroxysmal crying and 'pulling up' of the legs
- ○ B It peaks between 3 and 6 months
- ○ C It is due to cow's milk allergy
- ○ D There is no effective medical treatment
- ○ E It may require hospital admission

3.33 Regarding urinary tract infection (UTI)

- ○ A It is more common in boys in the first month of life
- ○ B *E. coli* is responsible in approximately 80% of cases
- ○ C Most UTIs are haematogenous in origin in neonates
- ○ D Significant bacteriuria occurs with > 103 CFU (colony-forming units) of bacteria/ml
- ○ E VUR is found in approximately 35% of children with a UTI

3.34 Regarding generalised tonic-clonic epilepsy

- ○ A Onset is generally after 5 years of age
- ○ B It is not associated with an aura
- ○ C The EEG may be normal between seizures
- ○ D After 15 years approximately 80% remain 'fit-free' off treatment
- ○ E First-line treatment is carbamazepine

3.35 NAI should be suspected if

- ○ A parents attend A&E immediately
- ○ B parents are over-protective
- ○ C a fractured tibia is seen in a 6-month-old infant
- ○ D the child has a depressed skull fracture
- ○ E the child has bilateral black eyes

3.36 With regard to adoption

- ○ A The adopted child takes on the nationality of their adoptive parents
- ○ B Applicants must be aged 18 or over
- ○ C The natural parents must give their informed consent before the adoption can proceed
- ○ D The child must live with the adoptive parents for 6 months before the order is finalised
- ○ E At age 16 an adopted child is entitled to their original birth certificate

3.37 Regarding rickets

- ○ A It is associated with epilepsy
- ○ B It may be secondary to ulcerative colitis
- ○ C It causes both genu valgum and genu varum
- ○ D Vitamin D-resistant rickets is an autosomal dominant condition
- ○ E It is associated with swelling at the wrists and costochondral junctions

3.38 Causes of generalised lymphadenopathy include:

- ○ A Sarcoidosis
- ○ B Kawasaki disease
- ○ C Phenytoin therapy
- ○ D Eczema herpeticum
- ○ E Juvenile chronic arthritis

3.39 Poor prognostic features of acute lymphoblastic leukaemia include:

- ○ A Age $<$ 2 years
- ○ B Age $>$ 10 years
- ○ C Being Caucasian
- ○ D Male sex
- ○ E Presenting WCC $>$ 20, 000/mm^3

3.40 Regarding inflammatory bowel disease

- ○ A Both Crohn's and ulcerative colitis are associated with finger clubbing, anaemia, erythema nodosum and arthritis
- ○ B Crohn's disease has increased over the past 20–30 years and now affects about 5 per 10, 000 individuals
- ○ C Ulcerative colitis is characterised by inflammation of the whole thickness of the bowel wall, especially the terminal ileum and proximal colon
- ○ D The 'string sign', 'skip lesions' and 'rose thorn ulcers' are characteristically seen in Crohn's disease following a barium meal and follow through
- ○ E Surgery is always required in the management of ulcerative colitis

3.41 Precocious puberty

- ○ A is defined as the onset of sexual maturation before 10 years in a girl
- ○ B is associated with McCune–Albright syndrome
- ○ C results in an increased final height
- ○ D is commonly associated with intracranial tumours in boys
- ○ E is associated with coeliac disease

3.42 Regarding bow legs (genu varum)

- ○ A They are normal in infants and usually correct by 5 years of age
- ○ B They may be secondary to osteogenesis imperfecta
- ○ C When due to 'medial tibial torsion', they are associated with bowing of the tibia which usually requires surgical correction
- ○ D They may be secondary to poliomyelitis
- ○ E They may be secondary to Osgood–Schlatter's disease

3.43 A normal 18-month-old infant

- ○ A can balance on one foot for a second
- ○ B can kick a ball forward
- ○ C can walk upstairs holding on, one foot per step
- ○ D can walk backwards
- ○ E may not be walking if a 'bottom-shuffler'

3.44 With regard to HIV infection

- ○ A The risk of vertical transmission in Europe is approximately 50%
- ○ B Breast-feeding should be avoided in developed countries
- ○ C It is a notifiable disease
- ○ D Pneumovax is contraindicated
- ○ E Testing for HIV antibodies helps to exclude neonatal congenital infection

3.45 A normal 3-year-old child

- ○ A can lace up their own shoes
- ○ B will play interactive games (eg tag) with other children
- ○ C is not yet capable of imaginary play
- ○ D is 'dry' by day, but seldom at night
- ○ E is able to dress themselves without supervision

EXTENDED MATCHING QUESTIONS

3.46 Theme: Respiratory distress in the newborn

A Congenital cystic adenomatous malformation
B Congenital diaphragmatic hernia
C Congenital pneumonia
D Meconium aspiration syndrome
E Persistent pulmonary hypertension of the newborn
F Pneumothorax
G Pulmonary haemorrhage
H Pulmonary hypoplasia
I Surfactant deficient lung disease (hyaline membrane disease)
J Transient tachypnoea of newborn

For each of the following scenarios please choose the most likely diagnosis from the above list. Each item may be used once or not at all.

1 An infant born at 24 weeks' gestation who has respiratory distress at birth.

2 An infant is born at 33 weeks' gestation with profound respiratory distress. Antenatal history reveals that there was rupture of membranes at 16 weeks, and the mother has been on erythromycin.

3 A baby is born by elective caesarean section at term (for breech presentation) following an uncomplicated pregnancy. At 15 minutes of age the baby is noted to be grunting.

3.47 Theme: Genetic diseases

A Autosomal dominant
B Autosomal dominant with incomplete penetrance
C Autosomal recessive
D Autosomal recessive with incomplete penetrance
E Lionised X linked
F Robertsonian translocation
G Sporadic
H Uniparental disomy
I X-linked dominant
J X-linked recessive

For each of the following conditions please choose the most appropriate mode of inheritance from the above list. Each item may be used once or not at all.

1 Achondroplasia.

2 Sickle cell disease.

3 Duchenne muscular dystrophy.

questions

3.48 Theme: Blood disorders

A Acute lymphoblastic leukaemia
B Aplastic anaemia
C β-thalassaemia intermedia
D Christmas disease
E G-6-PD deficiency
F Haemophillia A
G Henoch–Schönlein purpura
H Immune-mediated thrombocytopenia purpura
I Meningococcal septicaemia
J Sickle cell disease

For each of the following cases please choose the diagnosis that best fits the clinical and laboratory information from the above list. Each item may be used once or not at all.

1 A 4-year-child of eastern Mediterranean origin presents pale and tired following a upper respiratory illness treated with antibiotics. Her FBC reveals Hb 4.2 g/dl, WCC 12 × 10^9/l, plts 332 × 10^9/l, reticulocytes 6%.

2 A 6-year-old child develops a petechial rash. Her FBC shows Hb 11 g/dl, WCC 2.4 × 10^9/l, plts 9 × 10^9/l. A bone marrow trephine shows increase in megakaryocytes.

3 A 9-year-old child is febrile but well, and develops a purpuric rash on his lower limbs. His FBC shows Hb 13 g/dl, WCC 12 × 10^9/l (neutrophils 2 × 10^9/l, lymphocytes 10 × 10^9/l), plts 540 × 10^9/l. Coagulation coagulation profile: INR 1.2, acitvated partial thromboplastin time (APTT) 28 seconds, prothrombin time (PT) 11 seconds.

3.49 Theme: Infant nutrition

A 2 months
B 4 months
C 7 months
D 9 months
E 1 year
F 18 months
G 2 years
H 3 years
I 4 years
J 5 years

For each of the following foodstuffs please choose the most appropriate age for their introduction (in a normal infant) from the above list. Each item may be used once or not at all.

1 Pasta.

2 Baby rice.

3 Pureed meat and vegetables.

3.50 Theme: Systemic diseases

A Behçet's disease
B Dermatomyositis
C Kawasaki's disease
D Lyme disease
E Pauci-articular juvenile idiopathic arthritis
F Poly-articular juvenile idiopathic arthritis
G Rheumatic fever
H Septic arthritis
I Still's disease
J SLE

For each of the following case scenarios please choose the most likely diagnosis from the above list. Each item may be used once or not at all.

1 A 3-year-old boy has had a fever for 6 days, has swollen hands, conjunctivitis and cracked lips. Investigation reveals: CRP 67, ESR 40, Hb 12.1 g/dl, WCC 16 × 10^9/l (neutrophils 7 × 10^9/l, lymphocytes 8 × 10^9/l), plts 480 × 10^9/l.

2 A 12-year-old girl presents with feeling unwell, lethargy and pain in her knees and legs. On examination she is febrile (37.7°C), and has an erythematous rash on the face, particularly the eyelids. Investigations show: ESR 50, normal FBC, CK 700 IU/l.

3 A 7-year-old girl presents with pain in both knees, left ankle and right wrist. On examination, the joints involved are swollen, tender and have limitation of range of movement. Investigations show CRP 35, ANA +ve, Rheumatoid factor –ve, dsDNA antibodies –ve, anti-streptolysin O test (ASOT) –ve.

3.51 Theme: Genetic syndromes

A Achondroplasia
B Beckwith–Wiedemann
C Down's syndrome
D Fragile X syndrome
E Noonan's syndrome
F Patau's syndrome
G Pierre Robin syndrome
H Prader–Willi syndrome
I Rubenstein–Taybi syndrome
J Turner's syndrome

For each of the following cases please choose the diagnosis that best fits with the clinical features from the above list. Each item may be used once or not at all.

1 A term baby is noted to have a cleft palate and small chin. She appears to have problems breathing when placed supine.

2 A 4-year-old boy is having problems keeping up academically with his peers. On examination his neck is mildly webbed, and he has low-set ears.

3 A 6-year-old boy has marked behavioural problems. On examination he has large ears and a high forehead.

3.52 Theme: Vaccinations

A Acellular pertussis vaccine
B Conjugate pneumococcal vaccine
C Hepatitis A vaccine
D Hepatitis B vaccine
E Influenza vaccine
F Palivizumab (anti-RSV immunoglobulin)
G Ribavirin
H Salk polio vaccine
I Single measles vaccine
J Unconjugated pneumococcal vaccine

For the following situations please choose one vaccine that should be used instead of, or in addition to, the routine scheduled vaccines from the above list. Each item may be used once or not at all.

1 An ex-premature baby is now 2 months old. He has received his first DPT/HiB/Men C vaccine, but is still an inpatient on SCBU.

2 An 12-week-old infant is due for his routine immunisations; however, he had a prolonged episode of inconsolable crying after the previous set.

3 A 1-year-old infant has a splenectomy following a road traffic accident.

3.53 Theme: Psychiatric disorders

A Anorexia nervosa
B Asperger's syndrome
C Attention deficit-hyperactivity disorder
D Autism
E Depression
F Factitious Illness
G Psycho-social deprivation
H Post-traumatic stress disorder
I Rett's syndrome
J Temper tantrums

For each of the following cases please choose the most likely diagnosis from the above list. Each item may be used once or not at all.

1 A 3-year-old boy is brought to you, as his mother is concerned about his attention span. You note that he has very poor eye contact and poor verbal skills (having only a four-word vocabulary). His weight and height are appropriate for his age.

2 A 4-year-old girl is referred for speech therapy as she speaks very little. She has not had her MMR or pre-school boost. She appears withdrawn and shy but will play games if encouraged. Her weight is on the 2nd centile for her age (2 years ago was on 50th). Her dentition is poor.

3 An 11-year-old girl is confrontational at home and argues with her parents. She enjoys going out with her friends. Her school performance is falling and her concentration is poor. She has had thoughts of deliberate self-harm in the past and presents with some superficial lacerations to her left wrist. Taking a detailed history you elicit that she was sexually assaulted by a family friend 1 year ago.

3.54 Theme: Special investigations

A Angiography
B Bone scan
C CT
D Echocardiogram
E Electrocardiogram
F Electroencephalogram
G Magnetic resonance imaging (MRI)
H Plain X-ray
I Positron emission tomography
J Ultrasound

For each of the following clinical problems please choose the most useful investigation from the above list. Each item may be used once or not at all.

1 A 2-year-old boy is diagnosed and treated for Kawasaki's disease. You are concerned about possible complications and wish to investigate this.

2 A 1-year-old infant falls from a chair and hits her head on the concrete floor. She has a brief (1 minute) seizure 4 hours later

3 A 4-year-old child is febrile and is limping, complaining of pain in her left leg. There is some cellulitis overlying her distal left tibia.

BEST OF FIVE QUESTIONS

3.55 A 9-month-old infant presents with vomiting and crying. On examination she is afebrile and has a diffusely tender abdomen. No masses are palpable. Which one of the following diagnoses is the most important to exclude?

- A Gastroenteritis
- B Intussusception
- C Mesenteric adenitis
- D Hirschsprung's disease
- E Colic

3.56 A 9-month-old infant presents with coryzal symptoms and a hoarse barking cough. Select the most likely causative agent from the list below.

- A Adenovirus
- B *Haemophilus influenzae* tybe b
- C Parainfluenza virus type 3
- D Parvovirus
- E *Corynebacterium*

3.57 A 7-week-old baby boy is referred with a 2-week history of vomiting. He is being formula fed 5 oz (approximately 150 ml) every 2–3 hours. On examination he is well, thriving and has a normal examination. The most likely diagnosis is:

- A Pyloric stenosis
- B Gastro-oesophageal reflux
- C Over-feeding
- D Gastro-enteritis
- E Jejunal stenosis

questions

3.58 Which of the following is the first sign of puberty in boys?

- ○ A Growth spurt
- ○ B Pubic hair development
- ○ C Deepening of the voice
- ○ D Increase in testicular volume
- ○ E Axillary hair development

3.59 You diagnose a 7-year-old girl as having a generalised chest infection. Her respiratory rate is 30, $Sa(O_2)$ 98% in air, there is no recession. What would be the most appropriate course of action?

- ○ A Admit for intravenous antibiotics
- ○ B Allow home but arrange for intravenous antibiotics to be given by the home care nurses
- ○ C A 7-day course of oral amoxicillin
- ○ D A 7-day course of oral erythromycin
- ○ E Admit for oral antibiotics

3.60 A 3-year-old, fully immunised child presents with fever and difficulty in breathing. She has had tonsillitis over the past week. On examination she looks unwell, has mild recession, and a soft stridor is audible. What is the most likely diagnosis?

- ○ A Retro-pharyngeal abscess
- ○ B Bacterial tracheitis
- ○ C Epiglottitis
- ○ D Severe croup
- ○ E Fulminant pneumonia

3.61 A 13-year-old girl attends her GP surgery wanting to be prescribed the oral contraceptive pill (OCP). She is sexually active but does not want her mother to know (despite reasoning). Which of the following would be the most appropriate course of action?

- ○ A Refusal to prescribe as she is under the age of informed consent
- ○ B Prescribe her the OCP as it would be in her best interests
- ○ C Prescribe her the OCP if she meets the Gillick criteria
- ○ D Prescribe her the OCP on the condition that she gets parental consent
- ○ E Refuse to prescribe as this would condone under-age sexual intercourse, which is illegal

3.62 A 18-month-old infant who has an URTI presents with a convulsion. Which of the following features best fits with a typical febrile convulsion?

- ○ A One minute of left arm shaking followed by 6 minutes of tonic-clonic movement of all four limbs
- ○ B Eyes rolling back followed by a 3-minute generalised tonic-clonic seizure. Drowsy afterwards for 1 hour
- ○ C Going vacant and unresponsive for 2 minutes. Back to normal self afterwards
- ○ D A 25-minute generalised tonic-clonic seizure terminated with iv lorazepam
- ○ E A 5-minute generalised tonic-clonic seizure. Drowsy afterwards then a further 15-minute generalised tonic-clonic seizure

questions

3.63 You are called to counsel a woman in premature labour at 23/40. Which one of the following is the most appropriate information to give initially?

- A Unfortunately at this gestation there is 10–20% survival of which 50% will have some degree of handicap
- B Unfortunately at this gestation there are the following survival and handicap statistics (*tell her the figures for your own unit*)
- C Survival at this gestation is generally poor, and survivors may have long-term problems – (*then discuss with her the option of not resuscitating if the baby is in a poor condition*)
- D Babies at this gestation are very immature and will have a long and difficult time in the neonatal intensive care (*then discuss the likely problems and interventions that may be necessary*)
- E Babies at this gestation are extremely early and often do not survive but we will do everything we can

3.64 Which one of the following language milestones would you expect a normally developing 2-year-old child to have most recently acquired?

- A Six-word vocabulary
- B Greater than 100-word vocabulary
- C Three-word phrases
- D Tuneful babbling
- E Singing nursery rhymes

3.65 A 2-day-old 28/40 gestation neonate has a right-side intraventricular haemorrhage with no ventricular dilatation while on the ventilator. Which one of the following is the best advice to give to the parents?

- ○ A There are likely to be no significant long-term effects
- ○ B There should be no significant long-term effects provided that the ventricle doesn't dilate
- ○ C There may be some mild impairment of the left arm/leg
- ○ D There may be some very mild concentration difficulties in childhood
- ○ E It is probable that there will be no significant long-term effects but his development will be closely followed just in case

3.66 A 13-year-old boy develops gynaecomastia and comes to you as he is concerned. He reveals that he is being bullied at school as a result. What is the most appropriate course of action?

- ○ A Referral to a paediatric surgeon for consideration of surgical reduction of the breast tissue
- ○ B Arrange for assessment of the hypothalamic–pituitary axis
- ○ C Reassure him that this is physiological and a normal part of puberty
- ○ D Reassure him and arrange for clinical psychology support
- ○ E Reassure him and contact the school (with his consent) about the bullying

3.67 Which of the following is the most appropriate treatment for the contacts of a child who is admitted with meningococcal sepsis?

- A Treat all family members with rifampicin
- B Treat close contacts with rifampicin
- C Treat those contacts as advised by the Consultant for Communicable Disease Control (CCDC)
- D Treat close paediatric contacts with penicillin and adults with rifampicin
- E Leave the contact tracing and treatment to CCDC

3.68 Which one of the following is the best method of vascular access in a 5-year-old child brought into A&E resuscitation in asystole?

- A Peripheral venous cannulation
- B Femoral venous central line insertion
- C Long saphenous venous cannulation
- D External jugular central line insertion
- E Tibial intra-osseous needle insertion

3.69 A 2-year-old presents with a very painful scrotum. On examination the scrotum is swollen and inflamed on the right side. The testis on the right is not swollen though it is tender at the upper pole. What is the most likely diagnosis?

- A Testicular torsion
- B Idiopathic scrotal oedema
- C Torted hydatid of Morgagni
- D Epididymo-orchitis
- E Mumps orchitis

3.70 A 6-year-old complains that his foreskin balloons when he passes urine. On examination you note non-retractile foreskin with some preputial adhesions. What is the best course of action?

- ◯ A Advise gentle retraction of the foreskin in the bath
- ◯ B Advise that it can be normal at this age and should be left alone
- ◯ C Advise applying 1% hydrocortisone cream bd for 1/52
- ◯ D Refer for circumcision
- ◯ E Send a preputial skin swab for microscopy, culture and sensitivity

3.71 A 7-year-old girl has had two generalised tonic-clonic seizures (each lasting 7 minutes). The EEG shows epileptiform activity. Which one of the following is the most appropriate first-line anticonvulsant?

- ◯ A Phenytoin
- ◯ B Carbamazepine
- ◯ C Lamotrigine
- ◯ D PR diazepam (prn)
- ◯ E Sodium valproate

3.72 An 18-month-old infant girl with eczema is on the following treatment regimen: Oilatum in baths; 'baby' shampoo and soap; aqueous cream to affected areas qds. Mother uses 'non-biological' washing powder. On examination her skin is erythematous, excoriated and lichenified over the knees, thighs and flexor surfaces of the elbows. Which one of the following would be the next best step?

- ○ A Use aqueous cream instead of soap, advise using a greasier emollient and try an antihistamine at night
- ○ B Use 1% hydrocortisone to affected areas and continue with other measures
- ○ C Use emollient wet wraps at night for 1 week then continue current treatment
- ○ D Use fusidic acid-hydrocortisone to the affected areas for 1 week then continue current regimen
- ○ E Advise mother to continue current treatment and to try to exclude dairy products from the diet

3.73 An 8-month-old infant had a confirmed UTI at age 5 months and is currently on prophylactic antibiotics. A renal USS at the time of the UTI showed left renal pelvi-calyceal dilatation. What is the most appropriate investigation to perform next?

- ○ A Repeat renal tract USS
- ○ B Micturating cystourethrogram
- ○ C DMSA (dimercaptosuccinic acid) scan
- ○ D MAG-3 scan
- ○ E Repeat urine for MC&S (microscopy, culture and sensitivity)

3.74 A 9-year-old child has a large, swollen, fluctuant left submandibular lymph node. You notice that there is gross caries in most of her teeth. There is a buccal swelling adjacent to her lower left 'E' (primary molar). What is the best course of action?

- ○ A Course of oral amoxicillin and metronidazole and referral to her general dental practitioner (GDP)
- ○ B Admission for iv amoxicillin and metronidazole
- ○ C Referral to maxillofacial surgery for incision and drainage (I&D)
- ○ D Trial of oral antibiotics and surgical referral if no improvement after 5 days
- ○ E 5/7 course of iv ceftriaxone administered at home by community nurses, with review after the course
- ○ E Discharge her for GP follow-up

PAPER 1 ANSWERS

Multiple Choice Answers

1.1 AE

Pyloric stenosis has an incidence of 4 per 1000 live births with boys being affected more than girls in a ratio of 4:1. Approximately 15% of affected infants have a positive family history, mainly on the mother's side. Vomiting occurs after feeds and is projectile but not bile stained, since the obstruction is so high. Persistent vomiting leads to hyperchloraemic, hypokalaemic alkalosis needing fluid replacement with 0.9% normal saline plus added potassium.

Examination may reveal an olive-shaped abdominal mass during a test feed and an USS is the investigation of choice. A barium meal is also useful, although seldom required, and may be associated with an increased risk of aspiration. Treatment is surgical by Ramstedt's pyloromyotomy.

1.2 AE

The features of nephrotic syndrome include proteinuria, hypo-albuminaemia, generalised oedema and hyperlipidaemia. The serum albumin should be < 25 g/l with proteinuria > 1 g/m^2 per 24 hours.

Peak incidence is between 2 and 5 years of age with the majority being due to 'minimal change glomerulonephritis'. This accounts for 70–80% of cases of primary nephrotic syndrome. It has an incidence of approximately 2 in 100, 000 in the UK with a male:female ratio of 2:1. Over 90% respond to steroid therapy. Diffuse proliferative glomerulonephritis accounts for approximately 10% of cases of primary nephrotic syndrome (focal segmental 10%; membranous 2%). Other causes of nephrotic syndrome include congenital and secondary causes (eg collagen disorders, diabetes mellitus, toxins).

Initial management involves hospital admission for assessment and initiation of treatment. This may include corticosteroids, antibiotics, fluid management and diuretics. A high-protein, no salt-diet is poorly tolerated and a normal balanced diet provides adequate proteins. Salt restriction is only used if there is progressive oedema.

1.3 DE

LBW babies are those weighing < 2500 g, whereas very low birth weight (VLBW) babies weigh < 1500 g. Together they account for approximately 1 in 15 infants born in the UK. An LBW infant may be SGA, ie < 10th centile, premature, ie born before 37/40, or both.

SGA babies may reflect maternal factors, such as chronic illness (eg chronic renal failure (CRF)), hypertension, smoking, alcohol and undernutrition which results in placental insufficiency and thus intra-uterine growth retardation (IUGR). Maternal diabetes typically results in large for dates babies, but can also result in small for dates babies.

Problems include an increased incidence of congenital malformations, intrapartum asphyxia, hypoglycaemia, impaired thermoregulation, respiratory distress syndrome in premature infants and jaundice. Survival has improved over the years with over 95% of infants born weighing 2000–2500 g surviving and only about 8% of surviving infants suffering a major handicap (eg cerebral palsy).

1.4 CE

The indications for tonsillectomy include recurrent febrile convulsions associated with attacks of follicular tonsillitis, over three attacks of bacterial tonsillitis in two consecutive years and tonsils that are so grossly enlarged between infections that they meet in the midline causing stridor or sleep apnoea. Primary post-operative haemorrhage occurs within 24 hours and is usually due to inadequate haemostasis, whereas secondary haemorrhage occurs between 7 and 10 days and is commonly due to infection. Purulent follicular exudate may occur in both bacterial and viral tonsillitis. Some authorities claim that bacterial infection requires at least 10 days of antimicrobial treatment, although there is little evidence for this in industrialised societies.

Adenoidectomy is a useful treatment for glue ear, as the adenoids may encroach upon the nasopharyngeal orifice of the eustachian tube. It can be performed at the same time as grommet insertion and myringotomy.

1.5 C

Seventy-five per cent of children with autism are male and it usually develops before 3 years of age. Typical features of autism include: global impairment of language and communication; impairment of social relationships, especially empathy; and ritualistic and compulsive phenomena. All three features should be present to make a diagnosis. The 'idiot savant' is a rare feature of autism, the majority of children have decreased IQ.

The treatment of autism includes: educational and behavioural modification programmes; parental support and guidance; drugs such as tranquillisers, which may be needed to control panic attacks and sleep disorders, whereas haloperidol may be used to reduce stereotypes. Finally, residential placement may be necessary in severe cases where families are unable to cope; indeed up to 60% need long-term hospital or institutional care.

1.6 BCE

Vulvovaginitis is the commonest gynaecological disorder in girls. Commonly isolated organisms in pre-pubertal girls include *Gardnerella*, *Bacteroides* and streptococci. Threadworms may also cause symptoms and a vaginal foreign body should be considered if the discharge is bloodstained or offensive. Risk factors of infection include the lack of labial fat pads protecting the vaginal orifice and lack of the protective acid secretions found during the reproductive years.

Treatment includes: antibiotics if a specific organism is present; exclusion of an underlying cause, eg recent broad spectrum antibiotics; attention to vulval hygiene and avoidance of irritants and topical dienestrol cream in refractory cases which may help to clear infection by improving acidity. If the symptoms are not persistent, and in the absence of any other physical or behavioural signs, it is wiser not to discuss the possibility of sexual abuse with the mother, unless she expresses concern.

1.7 BE

Routine blood pressure measurement in children is not part of a screening test but should be done during the cardiovascular examination if indicated (ie in the presence of a cardiac murmur, history of renal/endocrine disease, malignant hypertension and family history (eg phaeochromocytoma)) or if there are signs of malignant hypertension (eg papilloedema), renal or adrenal masses, renal artery bruit, goitre, radio-femoral delay and neurofibromatosis found on examination.

The correct cuff size is approximately 2/3 the length of the upper arm. The 5th Korotkoff sound is often not heard in childhood, therefore K4 is used until adolescence, when K5 is used. In infants it is easier to use ultrasound Doppler or more typically 'Dinamap'. Results can be checked against a graph of normal values for age.

Secondary hypertension is more common in younger than in older children. After 13 years 50% is due to primary hypertension and 50% is due to secondary hypertension (of which 80% is due to renal parenchymal disease, 10% renal vascular disease and 10% 'other'). The level of hypertension requiring treatment is not really known but most clinicians treat a diastolic blood pressure > 90 mmHg before 13 years and > 100 mmHg after 13 years. NB Three or so recordings should be taken some weeks apart (in general) before a diagnosis of hypertension is made.

1.8 BE

If an infant suffers a cot death it is important to ensure the health of all siblings, especially the surviving twin, who is at increased risk and should always be admitted for observation, full septic screen and possible investigations for inherited metabolic disorders. Other risk factors include viral infections, hyperthermia (from over-wrapping/prone sleeping position), old PVC mattresses and parental smoking; indeed parents who stop smoking have been shown to significantly decrease the risk of their child suffering a cot death.

Apnoea monitors do not decrease the incidence of cot death and their use is controversial. Advantages include reassurance, ease of use and portability. However, they are expensive and often lead to false alarms and increased anxiety. They do not detect hypoxia and transcutaneous oxygen monitoring is under evaluation as an alternative. All parents issued with an alarm must be trained in basic life support. Parents should be taught to recognise and assess signs of illness in their babies and a system of increased surveillance by the health visitor and GP should be in place. Parents should be encouraged to consult their GP more readily and should not be criticised for it.

1.9 BD

More than 70% of acute bronchiolitis is due to RSV, the rest is secondary to adenovirus, rhinovirus, parainfluenza 1, 2 and 3 and influenza A. Nasopharyngeal aspirate leads to the detection of virus in secretions by immunofluorescence. Ribavirin is an antiviral agent of limited effectiveness against RSV, however, it is very expensive and difficult to administer and therefore treatment is usually only considered for 'high-risk' babies (eg premature infants, broncho-pulmonary dysplasia, congenital heart disease); the severely ill (PaO_2 < 8.6 or increased $PaCO_2$) or infants less than 6 weeks old. Salbutamol and theophylline have no effect on bronchiolitic obstruction in those under 1 year and there is limited evidence that ipratropium bromide is beneficial. Maternal IgG is protective against RSV.

1.10 ADE

Atopic eczema is very common, affecting up to 10% of children and its incidence is increasing. It generally occurs before 6 months, but can start at any age. Fifty per cent of cases have resolved by 5 years and 80% by 10 years. It may occur anywhere, but favours flexor surfaces in older children. Chinese herbal treatment has been shown to be effective, although its mechanism is unknown and adverse effects such as liver enzyme derangement are well documented. Initial treatment includes preventive measures such as avoidance of irritants and feeding high-risk infants with breast or hypoallergenic formula milks. Breast-feeding mothers may also consider avoiding consumption of common food allergens (eg cows' milk or eggs), though the evidence base for this is thin. Other more active treatment methods include skin emollients, topical steroids and antibiotics for secondary infection.

1.11 BDE

Truancy is associated with children over 8 years whereas school refusal commonly occurs in children between 5 and 11 years. They are typically from a small conventional social class I or II family who may collude over their child's non-attendance.

The prevalence is similar in boys and girls (truancy being more common in boys) and it commonly presents with various psychosomatic features.

1.12 ACDE

Causes of persistent snoring include hypertrophic nasal turbinates, allergic rhinitis, deviated nasal septum, nasal polyps, obesity and hypothyroidism. Recurrent tonsillitis may result in permanently enlarged tonsils which predispose to persistent snoring as do the macroglossia and other midfacial abnormalities associated with Down's syndrome.

1.13 AB

Eighty five per cent of infants with OA will have a tracheo-oesophageal fistula and 30% will have another abnormality. It may be part of the 'VACTERL' syndrome (ie Vertebral, Anorectal, Cardiovascular, Tracheo-oesophageal, Renal and Limb anomalies). Mothers typically have polyhydramnios antenatally.

It is diagnosed by the inability to pass a catheter into the stomach, which will be seen on X-ray to be coiled in the oesophagus. Contrast radiology should be avoided due to risk of aspiration. A tracheo-oesphageal fistula without an OA may present with recurrent pneumonia.

1.14 ABCD

The stepping reflex persists from birth to 6–8 weeks only.

1.15 AB

Treatment of cystic fibrosis includes regular (twice daily) chest physiotherapy and postural drainage which is essential in preventing and treating chest infections – the parents are usually taught to do this. A small number of children have had successful heart and lung transplants; however, donors are always limited and for most chronic patients surgery is not an option because of their poor general condition. Prophylactic flucloxacillin or other anti-staphylococcal antibiotics are helpful in avoiding staphylococcal chest infections, although there are conflicting opinions over the efficacy of this policy. Acute infections should be treated with 'best guess' antibiotics until cultures become available.

Patients have high-energy requirements and therefore need a high-calorie diet with normal protein and carbohydrate and high fat content. Fat restriction is no longer recommended as fat is the most energy-dense food. Supplemental pancreatic enzymes should be taken before all meals and snacks to prevent the clinical features of pancreatic insufficiency.

1.16 CE

Screening tests should have a high sensitivity (ie few false negatives) and high specificity (ie few false positives). Screening tests should be inexpensive; however, calculation of the true cost should include the money saved by detection of the disease at an early stage. Therefore 'cost-effective' is probably a more accurate term. The screening test should also be easy to perform, acceptable to the patient, repeatable and producing a yield of at least 1 in 10, 000 positive diagnoses of a treatable condition. Effective screening tests are available for a limited number of conditions. Ideally the defined condition screened for should be an important one with a recognisable latent or early symptomatic stage and a well-known natural history if untreated. Screening must be a continuous process to be effective and not a 'one-off'. Screening tests are ideally undertaken in primary care.

1.17 BCE

Migraines are generally preceded by an 'aura' that varies depending on which artery is affected. Vasoconstriction of a cranial artery may result in a transient oculomotor nerve palsy, ataxia, hemiparesis or aphasia. Intracranial pathology usually results in some permanent residual neurology. Migraine sufferers have a positive family history in 80% of cases, whereas acute severe headaches with no past medical or family history are more indicative of intracranial pathology. A significant space-occupying lesion may present with personality change, headaches that wake the child at night and are worse in the morning. Headaches may occur daily, escalating in a crescendo pattern; they may be accompanied by vomiting and a stiff neck and are exacerbated by coughing and bending over. 'Exclusion diets' are of no benefit and are generally part of the management of migrainous headaches, which should also respond to other simple measures such as lying in a darkened room, analgesics and antiemetics.

1.18 AC

Soto's syndrome (cerebral gigantism), Klinefelter's syndrome and Marfan's syndrome are all associated with tall stature.

1.19 ABD

Conditions that may result in a false-positive sweat test include Addison's disease, hypothyroidism, nephrogenic diabetes insipidus, glucose-6-phosphatase (G-6-PD) deficiency, mucopolysaccharidosis and ectodermal dysplasia. Bronchiectasis is a clinical feature of cystic fibrosis but will not cause a positive sweat test per se.

1.20 ADE

Part III of the Education Act 1993 is the UK legislation dealing with (SEN; it replaces the Education Act 1981). Its emphasis is on the earliest possible identification of SEN, including pre-school children and the importance of partnership between parents, children, schools, local education authorities (LEAs) and any other involved agencies. It aims to teach a wide and balanced curriculum, including the National Curriculum, and most children with SEN, including those with Statements, will have their needs met in mainstream schools.

Statements of SEN should be made and reviewed annually.

A child has a learning difficulty if he or she has a significantly greater difficulty in learning than the majority of children the same age or has a disability which either prevents or hinders the child from making use of educational facilities of a kind provided for children of the same age in schools within the area of the LEA. Special educational provision includes any educational provision that is additional to or different from that provided by mainstream schools for a child over 2 years or any educational provision given to a child under 2 years.

1.21 AD

Accidents are the single largest cause of death in children between 1 and 14 years and are responsible for approximately a third of all childhood deaths. Falls are the most common accident; however, road accidents (< 5% of all accidents) are the most common fatal accident accounting for about 50% of accidental deaths. Approximately 15% of all children per year attend A&E because of an accidental injury, the majority of these are boys aged 5–8 years from social classes IV and V.

1.22 ADE

Bilirubin toxicity is caused by free unconjugated bilirubin that is lipid soluble and therefore readily crosses brain cell membranes. Kernicterus is rare in term infants if the serum bilirubin does not exceed 380 mmol/l; however, premature infants or those with sepsis, hypoxia or acidosis may be affected at much lower levels. Symptoms include poor feeding, irritability, hypertonicity, opisthotonus, high-pitched cry, apnoea and convulsions.

Treatment involves phototherapy using narrow spectrum blue light of wavelength 450–475 nm, which causes photo-isomerisation and photo-oxidation of bilirubin to less lipophilic pigments. Management should also include ensuring adequate hydration and possible exchange transfusion. If the baby survives, long-term sequelae include choreoathetoid cerebral palsy, high frequency nerve deafness, paralysis of upward gaze and mental retardation.

1.23 ABCDE

All are safe to use during breast-feeding; however, thyroxine may interfere with neonatal screening for hypothyroidism.

1.24 ACDE

Nose picking is the most common cause of epistaxis in children, which is usually from the blood vessels on the nasal septum (Little's area). Other common causes include upper respiratory tract infections, allergic rhinitis and foreign bodies. Rarer causes include bleeding disorders and tumours of the nose and sinuses. Hypertension is a common cause of epistaxis in adults, but is rare in children.

1.25 CDE

There are 20 deciduous or 'milk' teeth and 32 permanent teeth (including four wisdom teeth). Teething may cause irritability, excessive salivation and a flushed appearance, but there is no fever. The first tooth to appear is generally a lower central incisor. Children do not have the hand-eye co-ordination to clean their teeth adequately until about 8–10 years of age, therefore parents should re-brush their children's teeth at least once a day. Thumb sucking may result in malocclusion and requires an orthodontic assessment.

1.26 AC

Infants with a UTI may present with vomiting, irritability and feeding problems. Between 2 and 5 years abdominal pain, fever, dysuria and frequency are classic, whereas school children have the more adult picture of dysuria, frequency, haematuria and loin pain, commonly without fever. Vesico-ureteric reflux is found in approximately 35% of children with a UTI. There is significant risk of progressive renal damage in the under-fives, thus prompt diagnosis and treatment is essential in children who should be investigated during or after their first UTI. Bacteria multiply rapidly at room temperature and should be 'plated' within 1 hour of collection. However, if this is not possible they may be refrigerated for up to 24 hours. Pyuria occurs in 50% of UTIs; however, there are other causes of pyuria including fever due to other causes, trauma, some drugs (eg diuretics), calculi and renal TB.

1.27 AD

Scabies is caused by the *Sarcoptes scabiei* mite which burrows into the skin to lay eggs. Typical sites include the interdigital webs and flexor aspects of the wrists of older children and adults; however, in infants the face and scalp are often involved as well. *Sarcoptes scabiei* is transmitted by close contact and has an incubation period of 2–4 weeks. Therefore, the whole family must be treated with γ-benzene hexachloride lotion on two occasions, 7 days apart to ensure eradication. Clothing and bedding should be decontaminated by hot washing.

Pruritus, which is usually worse at night, is due to sensitisation and persists for 4–6 weeks post eradication. Symptomatic measures such as calamine lotion or antihistamine should be tried and further re-treatment avoided as this will lead to irritant dermatitis and resistance.

1.28 ABCD

Orthopaedic complications of obesity include Blount's disease and slipped femoral epiphyses. Most obese healthy children are tall for their age with advanced bone age. If an obese child is short for their age it is important to exclude hypothyroidism, growth hormone deficiency, Cushing's, Down's and Prader–Willi syndromes.

1.29 ADE

The ketogenic diet is beneficial in some children with intractable seizures; however, it is unpalatable and difficult to enforce. Protective helmets should be worn while cycling; however, cycling (like swimming) must be supervised and busy/open roads avoided. It is also important that restrictions are kept to a minimum and education in mainstream schools the goal, with teachers kept informed about progress and drug treatment. Neurosurgery is indicated in a few, carefully selected children with refractory epilepsy.

1.30 ABDE

Hirschsprung's disease presents with constipation. It is due to a congenital absence of intestinal autonomic ganglion cells of the Auerbach and Messier plexus and is also associated with hypertrophy of extrinsic autonomic nerves. Causes of constipation include a low-fibre diet, over-enthusiastic potty training, anal fissures, anal trauma (eg post-operative, abuse), medication, dehydration, hypercalcaemia, hypothyroidism and spinal disorders (eg spina bifida).

1.31 BCDE

Phenylketonuria is an autosomal recessive condition with an incidence of 1:7000 in the UK. A heel prick blood test (the so-called Guthrie test) at day 6 looks for congenital hypothyroidism and can also detect elevated levels of phenylalanine. Phenylketonuria is associated with infantile spasms and will result in mental disability if the diagnosis is delayed and dietary restrictions not enforced. These restrictions should be continued until the child is at least 10 years old and ideally until adulthood. However, dietary restrictions should always be reinstated before conception and maintained throughout pregnancy to improve outcome, as genetically normal babies may be affected antenatally by the elevated levels of phenylalanine in the maternal circulation.

1.32 BCDE

1.33 AB

Acute lymphoblastic leukaemia is the leading paediatric malignancy and accounts for 85% of all childhood leukaemias. The peak incidence is between 2 and 6 years, with boys being slightly more affected than girls (55% versus 45%). Common presenting features include sepsis, lethargy, pallor, bleeding, bruising, petechiae, skeletal pain secondary to leukaemic infiltration, lymphadenopathy and hepatosplenomegaly. Investigations include a bone marrow aspiration and a blood film that reveals anaemia, thrombocytopenia and usually circulating blast cells. ALL is subdivided according to its immunological surface membrane markers, with 'common' having the best prognosis and 'B cell' the worst. Treatment involves ensuring good hydration, and allopurinol prior to chemotherapy in order to avoid renal impairment from urate stone formation. Epstein–Barr virus is associated with an increased incidence of developing Burkitt's lymphoma.

1.34 ABD

Spina bifida occulta is seen in 5–10% of all children and is usually found incidentally on X-ray. In meningocele the dorsal laminae are absent with a skin-covered lesion containing only cerebrospinal fluid (CSF) without underlying neurological involvement. Myelomeningocele is associated with neurological involvement. The neurological deficit depends on the level of the lesion, but double incontinence is the norm with paraplegia of the lower limbs. Both spastic and flaccid paralyses are seen, but the latter is more typical. In 90% of affected children hydrocephalus develops, which is most commonly secondary to an Arnold–Chiari malformation.

1.35 BD

The characteristic incubation periods for the following conditions are: chickenpox (10–24 days); measles (7–14 days); glandular fever (30–50 days); mumps (12–31 days); and rubella (14–21 days).

1.36 ADE

Antiepileptics taken antenatally increase the incidence of cleft lip and palate. Cleft lip should be repaired at 3 months, but cleft palate repair should be done between 6 months and 1 year. If surgery is performed during this time and the help of a speech therapist is enlisted, then speech has about a 75% chance of developing normally. Cleft palate may cause hearing loss due to the increased incidence of otitis media with effusion. Admission to SCBU should be avoided as this can hinder bonding. Special teats are available to use before surgical repair if feeding is problematical.

1.37 BE

The prevalence of asthma is increased in males, a personal or first-degree family history of atopy and amongst urban dwellers. Maternal smoking during pregnancy or passive smoking postnatally are also associated with an increased prevalence. Forceps delivery bears no relation to the risk of developing asthma, although a low birth weight is relevant.

1.38 ADE

Infantile spasms are rare with a usual onset between 4 and 9 months. They characteristically present with 'jack-knife' or 'salaam' attacks, which involve sudden flexion of the trunk, head and arms. These spasms typically last only a second but can recur several times a minute ('drop attacks' are characteristic of myoclonic astatic epilepsy). The EEG shows hypsarrhythmia in 66% and 70% will have localised or diffuse brain lesions on CT scan (tuberous sclerosis, brain malformations and chronic trauma), while 30% have no identifiable cause. The children with brain damage are refractory to treatment and develop psychomotor disabilities by 5 years, whereas cryptogenic cases respond better to treatment – seizures settle by 5 years and 50% develop a normal IQ. First-line treatment is prednisolone or ACTH for 3 months followed by benzodiazepines or valproate.

1.39 BD

No vaccine is contraindicated in cerebral palsy and full immunisation should be encouraged. Feeding difficulties occur due to hypertonia and problems arise because of the persistence of primitive reflexes (eg Moro, grasp and the asymmetric tonic neonatal reflexes).

1.40 ABC

There are certain common factors that predispose to child abuse. These include parental factors, such as coming from a broken home, and possibly being abused themselves and thus lacking a suitable role model from whom to develop good parenting skills. The parent may have a personality disorder or psychiatric illness. Risk factors associated with the child include prematurity, especially if the child was admitted to SCBU. The ensuing maternal separation results in a three-fold risk of abuse. Other features are children resulting from an unwanted pregnancy or those with a chronic illness or behavioural problems. The great majority of abused children are under 4 years old. Social factors are also an issue, any family crisis (eg bereavement, unemployment) increases the risk of abuse. Drug/alcohol dependence, poor housing, stepchildren, maternal exhaustion and social isolation are also all features. Extended family nearby lessens the risk.

1.41 ADE

Pica is defined as the 'eating of things that are not food'. It is likely to be associated with other signs of disturbed behaviour or a decreased IQ. If disciplinary approaches are unsuccessful a community paediatric referral may be appropriate to assess any developmental delay. It is associated with iron deficiency anaemia although it is not fully understood how or why, but may respond to a short course of iron supplements. The 'mouthing' of objects seen at 8 months is a normal transient developmental phase. However, if this persists beyond 2 years of age it is likely to be associated with some developmental problem.

1.42 BCDE

ADD is the term applied to unusually over-active children with accompanying lack of concentration, impulsiveness and emotional immaturity; boys are affected more than girls in a ratio of 5:1. Various associations include lead poisoning, drugs (eg phenobarbitone, phenytoin and theophylline) and possibly food additives (eg tartrazine-E102, sunset yellow-E110, carmoisine-E122 and amaranth). Other foods that may exacerbate hyperactivity in some children include cows' milk and wheat, though the evidence for this is weak. ADD is diagnosed more frequently in the USA. In the UK it is felt to be uncommon in isolation, but possibly occurs more frequently in association with conduct disorders or mental disability. Psychosocial assessment, which involves counselling parents and teaching simple behaviour modification techniques, is the mainstay of treatment. Medical treatment includes Ritalin and dietary advice may also have a role in a minority of children.

1.43 ABE

Salicylate poisoning can cause both respiratory alkalosis and metabolic acidosis. However, while respiratory alkalosis is a common finding in adults, children tend to have a more prominent metabolic acidosis. Hyperglycaemia, and hypoglycaemia, occur in salicylate poisoning. A serum salicylate level of < 400 mg/l is rarely symptomatic, whereas levels > 1.2 g/l are usually lethal. The mainstay of treatment involves correcting acidosis, hypoglycaemia and dehydration with intravenous (iv) fluid replacement, while ensuring a urine output of 5–6 ml/kg per hour. Urgent dialysis may be required for acute renal failure. Salicylate poisoning may also result in hypoprothrombinaemia, which can cause a coagulopathy requiring correction with vitamin K and FFP.

1.44 CDE

Tuberculin testing traditionally involves an injection into the flexor surface of the left forearm. The Heaf test is ideally read at 7 days (between 3 and 10 days) and the Mantoux test is read at 48–72 hours (but up to 96 hours). A positive result occurs when the area of induration is > 5 mm. NB the area of 'flare' is irrelevant.

The Heaf test is graded 0–4. Heaf grades 0–1 are negative and grades 2–4 are positive. Strongly positive reactions (ie Heaf grade 3–4 or induration > 15 mm) require further investigation and possible antituberculous chemotherapy.

1.45 ACDE

Sickle cell anaemia is an autosomal recessive condition that results from synthesis of an abnormal Hb chain (HbS). It is common among Blacks with 40% of black Africans and 10% of UK Afro-Caribbeans carrying HbS. It can be diagnosed by fetal blood sampling at around 18/40 or earlier by fetal DNA analysis of cells from amniotic fluid or trophoblast biopsy.

Heterozygotes (sickle cell trait) are usually asymptomatic unless severely hypoxic and typically have a normal haemoglobin and blood film. Homozygotes (sickle cell disease) however, present with acute haemolysis and frequent painful sickling crises of mainly fingers and toes from about 6 months, and larger joints from 3–4 years. Their haemoglobin is usually around 6–8 g/dl and their blood films typically show hypochromia, target cells, Howell–Jolly bodies and occasional sickle cells. The associated chronic haemolytic anaemia results in an increased incidence of pigment gallstones leading to biliary colic.

Management involves treating the underlying cause and supportive measures using fluids, oxygen and analgesia. Antibiotics, blood or even exchange transfusion may also be necessary acutely. Splenectomy should be considered for hypersplenism or recurrent sequestration crises and should always be covered with pneumococcal vaccination with or without prophylactic penicillin.

Answers to Extended Matching Questions

1.46 Analysis of blood gases

	Normal range
pH	7.35–7.45
$p(CO_2)$	4.5–5.5 kPa
$p(O_2)$	6.5–13.5 kPa
HCO_3	25–35 mmol/l
BE (Base excess)	–1 to +1 mmol/l

Table 1 Normal ranges of blood gas variables

Capillary samples – approximate normal ranges are as given in Table 1. However $PaCO_2$ upper limits can be allowed up to 6.5 kPa. Lower PaO_2 values can be permitted on venous samples, however, if oxygenation is the concern then an arterial sample should be taken (capillary samples are well arterialised and can be interpreted as arterial)

1 B – Compensated respiratory acidosis

The $PaCO_2$ is raised, but the pH is normal so this is a fully compensated gas. Given the history this is a compensated respiratory acidosis.

2 G – Partially compensated metabolic acidosis

7.32 is mildly acidotic, the likely diagnosis is diabetic ketoacidosis. The HCO_3^- is low therefore this is a metabolic acidosis, however the $PaCO_2$ is low (2.9) so there is some respiratory compensation (though NOT fully).

3 I – Respiratory acidosis

An alkalotic gas. The $PaCO_2$ is slightly raised, and there is a very raised HCO_3^-, this is consistent with a metabolic alkalosis. (The likely diagnosis in this child is pyloric stenosis or possibly a pre-ampullary duodenal stenosis – leading to loss of H^+ and Cl^- in the vomit.)

1.47 Vaccinations

1 G – Normal schedule with substitution of inactivated for live polio vaccine and no BCG

The 'Green Book' for immunisation against infectious disease states that children with HIV should receive the normal immunisation schedule, but not receive BCG and recommend the substitution of inactivated for live polio vaccine as the contacts of the child particularly may be immunocompromised.

2 D – Normal immunisation schedule with substitution of inactivated for live polio vaccine

Siblings of immunocompromised children (for example those receiving chemotherapy for ALL) should receive inactivated polio. Live polio vaccine is excreted in stools for 4–6 weeks after the dose is given.

3 C – Normal immunisation schedule

Children with sickle cell trait should receive the universal schedule. Those with sickle disease should receive both the conjugated pneumococcal vaccine with their standard 2, 3, 4 months vaccines and the unconjugated vaccine at 2–3 years.

1.48 Infant milk formulae

1 E – High-energy formula

The chronic lung disease means that the infant uses more calories to breathe and therefore has a higher than normal daily calorie requirement. A higher calorie formula is needed and a high-energy formula would be most appropriate. Pre-term formulae are more calorific but unsuitable for infants of this age.

2 A – Breast milk

In the UK, maternal HIV, current cytotoxic therapy or galactosaemia in the infant are the only medical reasons not to breast-feed.

3 F – Hydrolysed protein formula

The clinical scenario fits with a cow's milk protein intolerance. Gastro-oesophageal reflux is associated with cow's milk protein intolerance as a result of eosinophil infiltration in the oesophagus. Soya formulae are not recommended for infants under 6 months as they contain phyto-oestrogens.

1.49

1 J – Rolandic epilepsy

These features best fit with 'benign' Rolandic epilepsy. The age of onset and the type of seizure are typical. The centro-temporal spikes are diagnostic. The term 'benign' Rolandic epilepsy is slightly misleading in that, although the outcome is usually good with the seizures disappearing by adulthood, the nocturnal seizures are increasingly linked to SUDEP (sudden unexplained death in epilepsy). The risk of SUDEP lowers the threshold of many clinicians to start anti-epileptics.

2 A – Absence epilepsy

Absence seizures are often first noticed as 'poor concentration' at school. The child is concentrating but is having absences that may be mistaken for daydreaming. Classically, 3/s spikes on EEG are seen. In an outpatient setting hyperventilation is a useful stimulus to bring on a seizure, thus making the diagnosis.

3 B – Complex partial seizures (of the temporal lobe)

The prodromal features described, and the type of seizure described, are common in temporal lobe epilepsy.

1.50 Skin rashes

1 F – Pityriasis rosea

The presence of the single spot and then the development of this rash fits very well with the 'Herald' patch and 'Christmas tree' rash of pityriasis rosea. Pityriasis is probably viral in origin but the exact causative organism is unknown. The rash appears 1–2 weeks after the Herald patch, lasts 2 weeks then slowly resolves. Treatment is symptomatic.

2 A – Erysipelas

Slapped cheek syndrome is possible but this child is systemically unwell and the cheeks are cellulitic. Erysipelas is commonly caused by Group A streptococci. Treatment is with iv penicillin.

3 G – Rubella

Rubella has an incubation period of 2–3 weeks. The rash appears on the face, spreads down to the trunk and then finally affects the limbs. Cervical, occipital and posterior auricular lymph nodes are often enlarged before the appearance of the rash.

1.51 Renal diseases

1 G – Post-streptococcal glomerulonephritis

Red urine probably indicates haematuria. He is hypertensive and is having symptomatic headaches, these two features fit with a nephritis. A low C_3 and normal C_4 is typical for post-streptococcal glomerular nephritis.

2 E – Mesangial IgA nephropathy

Though he has had a recent URTI, the onset of the symptoms is too soon after the URTI for post-streptococcal glomerular nephritis (which is normally more than a week after). In addition his blood pressure is normal (which doesn't fit with a nephritis), and the complement levels are normal.

3 C – Haemolytic uraemic syndrome

Any renal impairment following a diarrhoeal episode should raise the suspicion of HUS. This is confirmed by a very high urea, low Hb and low platelets. Examination of a blood film would show a microangiopathic haemolytic anaemia. HUS is the most common cause of acute renal failure in childhood. It is caused by verotoxins produced by *Escherichia coli* O157 (a cause of bloody diarrhoea). Over half of the cases require dialysis.

1.52 The unwell infant

1 A – Cardiac failure

Difficulty completing feeds, along with sweating, is a good indicator of heart failure in infancy. Hepatomegaly is another sign of cardiac failure. It is important to distinguish between cardiac failure (not cyanotic and due to L→R shunt), and duct-dependent cardiac lesions (duct dependent – so when duct closes infant becomes cyanotic).

2 F – Galactosaemia

The features of hepatomegaly, jaundice and abnormal clotting go along with both sepsis and hepatitis due to galactosaemia. The urine-reducing sugars would be negative in sepsis – although in these cases in practice you would treat for sepsis as well.

3 I – Non-accidental injury

NAI, HDN (haemorrhagic disease of the newborn) and Group B streptococcal sepsis are the three main possibilities in this case. HDN is less likely as the baby is bottle-fed so should be getting sufficient vitamin K. If this were HDN then it would probably be an acute event, and the fact that the baby is 'always' crying points against this and more towards NAI.

1.53

1 I – Vitamin E

Ataxia and weakness are signs of vitamin E deficiency. Vitamin E is routinely supplemented in children with cystic fibrosis. This is because vitamin E is fat soluble (along with A, D and K) and may be malabsorbed due to exocrine pancreatic deficiency.

2 F – Vitamin B_{12}

Folic deficiency is unlikely in a vegan diet as green vegetables and legumes are good sources. Vitamin B_{12}, however, is mainly obtained from dairy products and meat products and deficiency results in megaloblastic anaemia. Treatment with B_{12} supplements stimulates a good bone marrow response.

3 H – Vitamin D

Vitamin D deficiency leads to reduced Ca^{2+} uptake from the gut. Ca^{2+} is resorbed (stimulated by PTH) from the bone to maintain serum levels. Alkaline phosphatase levels may be increased reflecting osteoblastic activity. Clinically this leads to rickets. There may be prominent wrists (due to the 'cupped, splayed, frayed' appearance of the radial and ulna metaphyses (and those of the other long bones)). A 'rachitic rosary' may be present due to swelling of the costochondral junctions. Treatment is with vitamin D supplementation.

1.54 Respiratory conditions

1 D – Foreign body inhalation

In a toddler who presents with difficulty in breathing foreign body aspiration must always be considered. Toddlers are inquisitive and will put most small objects in their mouths. Any asymmetry in expansion or wheeze should increase the index of suspicion.

2 G – Pertussis

An immunisation history must always be asked for (and the personal child health record ('red book') should be used). A cough that occurs in paroxysms, subconjunctival haemorrhages from repeated coughing and a marked lymphocytosis are all classic features of whooping cough. Treatment is supportive but erythromycin can be given to limit infectivity to other children. The cough can last up to 3 months (the 100 days cough).

3 B – Atopic asthma

A previous history of an atopic condition or a family history of atopy increases the risk of asthma (and other atopic conditions). A nocturnal cough is a recognised presentation of asthma in pre-school children. A trial of an inhaled bronchodilator via a spacer is worthwhile.

Best of Five Answers

1.55 D: Werdnig–Hoffman disease (spinomuscular atrophy type 1)

While Down's, Prader–Willi, and Beckwith–Wiedemann can all present with neonatal hypotonia it is not severe enough to cause respiratory insufficiency.

1.56 C: Check inhaler technique

The most important step to take is to check inhaler technique before going to the next stage of the British Thoracic Society (BTS) guidelines. If the current medication is not being effectively given then there is no point in increasing the medication.

1.57 E: Bronchiolitis

These are the clinical features of bronchiolitis – most frequently caused by RSV, but also adenovirus and influenza virus. These features do not really fit with croup. Viral-induced atopic wheeze is possible.

1.58 D: Only the mother can consent to the operation

If the parents are unmarried then the father has no legal parental responsibility. Although the law was changed this year to give parental rights to non-married fathers who appear on the birth certificate. Therefore only the mother can consent to procedures on the child. The child can consent for themselves once they are 'competent' (see Gillick competence on page 178 (3.61 answer)). It is very unlikely that a 10-year-old child would be competent to consent to an operation (appreciating the risks of anaesthesia). An important point is that even if a child can consent to a procedure when competent (if under 16), legally they cannot refuse one if the person with parental responsibility consents. However, as of December 2003 the law has changed so that the person named on the birth certificate **does** have parental responsibility (even if unmarried). This will not apply retrospectively – ie if a child is born before December 2003 then the father has no parental responsibility if not married to the mother.

1.59 B: Breast development

Breast development is the first sign of puberty in girls (from 8 years). Menarche occurs approximately 2 years later (at Tanner stage 4). Peak height velocity will usually coincide with menarche. There is a wide range in the times of onset of the stages.

A good reference for the sequence of development is: Marshall, W.A., and Tanner, J.M. 1969. Variations in pattern of pubertal changes in girls. *Archives of Diseases in Childhood*, **44** (235), 291–303.

1.60 A: Perthes' disease

As this child is afebrile septic arthritis and irritable hip are unlikely. Irritable hip is uncommon in this age group anyway (usually affecting those aged 1–4 years). Osgood–Schlatter's disease is pain due to inflammation of the patella tendon at the tibial insertion. SUFE occurs classically in adolescence (M:F 3:2).

1.61 D: Modification of healthcare systems to optimise patient care

This is the best interpretation of clinical governance. The other statements are all important 'pillars' (parts) of clinical governance but none encapsulate the concept in its own right.

1.62 D: Poor compliance

This is the only explanation that fits. In poor compliance the TSH rises as the thyroxine is repeatedly missed; however, when the child has to come for TFTs the thyroxine is restarted and so the plasma T_4 rapidly reverts to normal, but the TSH is slower to recover.

1.63 B: Advise her to try to exclude the suspected food and see if this produces an improvement in his symptoms – if so then reintroduce and see if the symptoms return.

Food intolerance is a difficult area, with parents wanting definitive tests and answers. The only scientific and practical way of 'detecting' an intolerance is to remove the suspected foodstuffs and see if there is an improvement in symptoms. A staggered reintroduction of individual foods can then be tried to see if the symptoms recur. RAST tests and skin prick tests have some limitations of both specificity and sensitivity and need to be interpreted in combination with the clinical history. A well, thriving child is less likely to have serious pathology (though you should always keep this in the back of your mind).

1.64 D: External angular dermoid

External angular dermoid is by far the most likely diagnosis. External angular dermoids (dermoid cysts) are embryological remnants that contain dermal and epidermal tissues. The site of the lump means that the other options are much less likely. Neurofibromas are not common in children this young.

1.65 B: Pulling to stand

Neurodevelopment is a dynamic process. Infants achieve 'milestones' gradually, as an example they do not suddenly sit unsupported one morning having been unable to the previous morning. There is an inherent variation in when a child will achieve a 'milestone', and it is important to know the range of ages at which it is normal to develop skills. The Denver II chart is a useful tool, which shows the normal progression of development and the ranges at which certain milestones occur. If a child has not achieved a milestone by the age at which 90% of the population would be expected to have achieved it, then further assessment may be indicated.

If a child is delayed in one of the neurodevelopmental areas then that may well affect the development of another area.

Sitting unsupported: by 8 months

Pull to stand: by 10 months

Rolling prone to supine: by 7 months (supine to prone 1 month later)

Climb up stairs without support: by 20 months

Transferring hand to hand: actually a fine motor milestone! (by 7 months)

NOTES ON DEVELOPMENTAL ASSESSMENT

Development is the maturation of the nervous system and is dependent on experience/stimulus. By the end of the second trimester the fetal brain has a full complement of nerves cells; however, neurodevelopment is the maturation of these cells and the development of connections between them.

Neurodevelopment is a dynamic process. Infants achieve 'milestones' gradually; for example, they do not suddenly sit unsupported one morning having been unable to the previous morning. There is an inherent variation in when a child will achieve a 'milestone', it is important to know the range of ages at which it is normal to develop skills. The Denver II chart is a useful tool in showing the normal progression of development and the ranges at which certain milestones occur. If a child has not achieved a milestone by the age at which 90% of children would be expected to have achieved it, then further assessment may be indicated.

If a child has delay in one of the neurodevelopmental areas then that may well affect the development of a different area.

Development depends on the stimulation to develop and, importantly, loss of primitive reflexes and development of acquired reflexes.

Remember the Areas of Development

- Gross motor
- Fine motor and vision
- Speech and hearing
- Social.

Gross motor

The gross motor skills develop in a 'cephalo-caudal' manner (from the head working downwards). This means that head control is one of the earliest gross motor milestones achieved and is usually followed by lifting of the shoulder when prone, and gradually getting better truncal control, sitting up, crawling then walking. Gross motor skills are very dependent on the loss of primitive reflexes and development of acquired reflexes. An infant will not be able to sit unsupported if the lateral saving reflex (putting arms out laterally to stop falling sideways) hasn't developed. Likewise if the parachute reflex (putting arms out in front to stop falling forwards) does not develop then a child will not be able to learn to walk unsupported.

Fine motor and vision

Development of fine motor skills is dependent on gross motor and postural development as well as good vision. During the first 6 months of life a child will visually fix and track an object but lacks the manipulative skills to grasp it. These manipulative skills develop so that by 18 months the child can accurately reach out and pick up a small object with a pincer grip.

Speech and hearing

Hearing is paramount in the development of normal speech and language skills. The most common cause of delayed speech is hearing problems – all children with delayed speech development must have a hearing test arranged soon. Infants recognise and respond to voice – by 8 weeks a baby should 'still' to their mother's voice. Over the first year an infant will learn noises and intonation and may not produce any words but may babble with mature intonation. 'Dada' is usually the first 'word' as the 'da' sound is easier to produce than a 'ma'. From 1 year the number of words increases with the child putting words together by 2 years.

Social

Human social behaviour and interaction is extremely complicated and needs to be learnt by a developing child. Initially a baby will produce a social smile by 8 weeks to all humans. Over the first year an infant will develop social interaction with all humans but towards the end of the first year will start to develop 'stranger awareness' and will be anxious when not in the presence of a carer they recognise. After the first year the child starts to develop personal social skills such as feeding, dressing and continence. The development of social and interaction skills continues throughout childhood and schooling.

Primitive Reflexes

Reflex	Age at onset	Disappearance
Rooting	Birth	9 months
Palmar grasp	Birth	Palm: 2–3 months foot: 7–8 months
Asymmetric tonic neck	1 month	3–5 months
Galant	Few days after birth	7–8 days
Moro	Birth	2–3 months
Hand opening	Birth	2–3 months
Stepping	4 days	2 months
Placing	4 days	5–9 months

Table 3 Summary of the primitive reflexes

1.66 E: Building a tower of two cubes

Casting of objects: by 5 months

Thumb and forefinger grasp: by 10 months

Banging two cubes together: by 11 months

Feed self with spoon: by 19 months

Build tower of two cubes: by 20 months

See neurodevelopmental milestones (page 214)

1.67 D: Admit for 24 hours of neurological observations

The National Institute for Clinical Excellence (NICE) have produced national guidelines for the management of head injuries. It is a little more complicated in children for a number of reasons. Children tend to vomit after injury, this may not be due to a significant brain injury but as a response to the injury. CT scanning (investigation of choice for significant head injuries) requires a degree of co-operation and lying still, which may be difficult for younger children (< 5 years). In this case where there was loss of consciousness and some post-event vomiting, a CT scan may be indicated. However, as the child is 3 years old this may be difficult unless it is performed under general anaesthetic. In these cases admission for neurological observation is preferable, if there is any decrease in GCS or development of focal neurological signs then a CT is definitely indicated.

1.68 D: Dada/mama (specific to person)

See neurodevelopmental milestones (page 214).

1.69 D: Pure tone audiometry

Pure tone audiometry is performed by placing headphones on the child and playing tones of various frequencies and intensities through them. The test requires a degree of co-operation, which should be present in a 5-year-old. Oto-acoustic emissions (measuring the sound 'echo' from the cochlear) are a useful screening test but cannot distinguish between conductive and sensory deficits. Brainstem-evoked responses (measuring brain wave response to auditory stimulus) can be performed at any age but is a lengthy test. The distraction test is routinely performed by health visitors at 8 months of age.

1.70 E: The birthmark may get larger until 2 years of age, and 70% resolve by 5 years and 95% by 10 years

This is indeed the natural course of a capillary haemangioma. It is important that parents are told that there is a chance that the birthmark may never completely resolve.

1.71 D: Anti-nuclear antibodies

All these investigations are useful when making the diagnosis. Once the diagnosis has been made, the investigation that has the biggest impact on management is ANA. There is a close correlation between being ANA +ve and development of iridocyclitis (which can lead to blindness). ANA +ve children must have close ophthalmological follow-up.

1.72 A: Basal–bolus regimen

The basal–bolus system involves a dose of long-acting insulin with three doses of short-acting insulin per day to coincide with meals, allowing greater flexibility with eating times and amounts (this is easier with older children). The long-acting insulin ensures a background level that provides more stable glycaemic control. This is ideally the best regimen for any diabetic child. However, a 3-year-old child is unlikely to conform to the 'set' three meals per day and will tend to 'graze' (ie take small frequent bits of food). Given this eating behaviour a regimen where there is a more constant level of insulin in the bloodstream is appropriate. Therefore, a twice-daily regimen is more likely to provide better control, indeed in some children whose eating patterns are so erratic a once-a-day injection of a long-acting insulin provides the best control.

1.73 D: Dietary iron deficiency

Iron deficiency is the most likely as there is a microcytic anaemia with a low serum ferritin. The most likely cause of this in the UK is a dietary deficiency. Chronic helminth infection is a common cause worldwide. Folate deficiency leads to megaloblastic anaemia. As the Hb electrophoresis shows 98% HbA (normal) then α-thalassaemia is ruled out.

1.74 E: Discharge home but arrange for daily review and FBCs

Since there is no 'mucosal' bleeding (ie lips/gums/tongue, urine or bowel) there is a lower risk of serious intracranial bleeding. There is no need to acutely treat the lower risk groups. The parents should have the diagnosis explained to them and the child should have frequent reviews. The natural course is that the average time to normal platelet numbers is one month, most others will be normal by six months but a small proportion will have chronic ITP. If there is evidence of mucosal bleeding then treatment is advisable.

PAPER 2 ANSWERS

Multiple Choice Answers

2.1 A

Below 16 years of age, consent of a parent or guardian is required, unless emergency treatment is required (when consent from a person *in loco parentis* is also unnecessary) or the child has given consent and the doctor considers that the child is of sufficient understanding to make an informed decision about medical care (including oral contraception) and the child refuses that the parents be asked.

If a child below 16 years of age refuses surgery it can still be carried out if the doctor believes the child doesn't have sufficient understanding to make an informed decision or if a court has considered the child's objection and told the doctor to proceed.

A mother and father have equal parental responsibilities for their legitimate child. If parents disagree it is probably inappropriate to proceed, although only one parent is needed for consent. An unmarried father is only financially responsible for his child, he has no intrinsic rights. (See answer 1.58.)

2.2 ACD

Acne affects 90% of teenagers and 25% of infants. Boys are more commonly affected than girls and it persists beyond the age of 25 in 15%. Acne is usually associated with normal levels of testosterone. Causes include medication (eg oral contraceptive pill, steroids, phenytoin), irritants (eg cosmetics), occlusion (eg friction by head bands), emotional stress, menstruation and endocrine abnormalities (eg Cushing's syndrome, diabetes, virilising tumour, polycystic ovaries).

Propionibacterium acnes is an anaerobic diphtheroid and this together with yeast colonises the blocked sebaceous glands and breaks down sebum releasing free fatty acids which cause an inflammatory reaction in the dermis. Secondary infection of papules causes pustules, cysts and scars.

In moderate cases, the treatment with erythromycin should continue for at least 6–12 months as its maximum effect is not achieved before 3–6 months. Even so, it may still relapse requiring a further 3 months of treatment, thus the patient must be well motivated. Severe cases (multiple cysts, pits, scars and keloids) and resistant moderate cases should be referred to the dermatologist. Roaccutane should only be prescribed by the hospital specialist. Liver function tests and lipids should be checked before starting treatment and monitored throughout. Roaccutane causes dry skin and mucosa and is 100% teratogenic (therefore oral contraception should be continued for at least one month after cessation of treatment).

2.3 ABE

A facial petechial rash may be a sign of smothering, although it may also be present in whooping cough. A generalised petechial rash, however, should raise suspicion of idiopathic thrombocytopenic purpura or meningococcal septicaemia. Multiple bruising on the shins of a 7-year-old boy is a normal finding, but bruising over the face, upper arms, wrists or inner thighs (with or without grip marks) in a child less than 9 months is of concern. A Mongolian blue spot is commonly mistaken for abuse, but is in fact a harmless congenital blue marking, frequently occurring over the buttocks and sacrum.

Other superficial features compatible with physical child abuse include bite marks, a torn fraenum (from, for example, forced bottle-feeding), lacerations, ligature marks, burns and scalds. Bony injuries include metaphyseal or epiphyseal fractures, which raise suspicion of a twisting or pulling injury. Also, multiple fractures at different stages of healing or delayed presentation of fractures need very careful assessment.

2.4 ACD

Turner's syndrome affects 1 in 2500 women. It has the genotype (XO) and mosaicism may occur with the genotype (XO, XX). NB testicular feminisation has the genotype (XY). Features apparent at birth include a webbed neck, low posterior hairline and widely spaced nipples. Other features include a 'shield-shaped' chest, coarctation of the aorta, left heart defects, cubitus valgus, short stature (less than 130 cm), hyperconvex nails, nystagmus, 'streak' ovaries – rudimentary or absent – and an association with Crohn's disease.

Somatotrophin is a useful treatment for short stature but only before the epiphyses have fused. Counselling is also an important part of the treatment and should cover genetic, medical and infertility issues.

2.5 BD

Molluscum contagiosum is a pox DNA virus infection that typically presents as small pearly umbilicated lesions anywhere on the body with characteristic satellite spread around the original lesion. The incubation period is 2–7 weeks and it spreads easily to siblings (eg via bath water) and the child remains infectious as long as the lesions are present. Atopic and immunocompromised children are particularly susceptible. The treatment of choice is patience as spontaneous resolution is the rule, typically after several months. Removal with phenol or liquid nitrogen is generally reserved for cosmetic reasons only.

2.6 BCE

Both irritant and contact dermatitis spare the flexures and should be treated by exposure to fresh air as much as is possible, frequent nappy changes, careful cleansing with baby lotion and routine use of barrier creams (eg zinc/castor oil). Secondary infection may be treated initially with a local antiseptic or antimicrobial. Candidiasis presents as a red rash with satellite lesions and shallow ulcers and lesions on the skin should be treated with antifungal cream and white oral/mucosal lesions with gel.

Nappy rashes do not commonly become secondarily infected with *S. aureus*. However, if there is impetiginous crusting or bullae, then it must be considered. Topical antibiotics may be sufficient treatment if the infection is localised to the nappy area. If nappy rash fails to settle with the use of emollients while bathing and aqueous creams afterwards, then 0.5–1% hydrocortisone may be applied to the face and intertriginous areas. Potent fluorinated steroids (ie Dermovate) should only be used on thicker areas for less than 2–4 weeks and only if treatment with mild-–moderate steroids has been unsuccessful.

Seborrhoeic dermatitis is an erythematous greasy rash which commonly involves the nappy area, the occipital region and behind the ears. It may become secondarily infected with *Candida* requiring treatment with antifungals.

2.7 ADE

Munchausen's by proxy refers to signs or symptoms in a child deliberately fabricated or induced by an adult. The child may be normal or have an illness and is usually of pre-school age. Although no organic cause can be found for the symptoms and all investigations are normal, the child may well show evidence of emotional abuse and/or failure to thrive. It is associated with a mortality of 2–10%.

The perpetrator is usually the mother, rarely the father, often with some kind of medical knowledge or training (eg nurse). She is generally not psychiatrically unwell, but often has a personality disorder with maladaptation in other areas. She may have been abused herself as a child and is now seeking the attention of carers or she may be seeking refuge from other problems. Confrontation with evidence, while involving the partner, is a key part of the management, and this should be done in a sympathetic manner. Management should be discussed with social services and a strategy or case conference should be organised to consider the child's welfare, who should stay with the family if at all possible. Further help should be offered in the form of counselling, psychiatric referral and family/ behavioural therapy.

2.8 AC

There is a male to female ratio of 2:1. The feet are held in equinovarus (ie downwards and inward) and club foot is associated with spina bifida. Initial management begins within 1 week of birth with splinting, where the deformity is 'over-corrected'. The infant then has weekly foot manipulations and if the foot has not corrected by approximately 3 months operative reduction or tendon release and fixation may be necessary.

2.9 BCE

Cleft palate is equally prevalent (and is increasing in incidence) in boys and girls. Cleft lip is more common in boys, affects 1 in 750 live births and is associated with cleft palate in approximately 50% of cases. The risk to a child with one affected sibling is 5% and with two affected siblings is 9%.

2.10 E

Tonsillectomy is indicated in children having more than four attacks of acute tonsillitis per year causing significant systemic illness, interference with growth, and school absences, recurrent cervical adenitis or peritonsillar abscess. It is associated with significant morbidity and mortality and should only be performed if clinically indicated and not at the request of the parents.

Although swallowing is uncomfortable, this does not lead to complete dysphagia post-operatively. Other complications include primary haemorrhage, occurring within 24 hours and usually due to an inadequately ligated/cauterised vessel, and secondary haemorrhage, which is commonly due to infection and occurs in 1% of patients approximately 1 week after the procedure. Quinsy (peritonsillar abscess) is a complication of tonsillitis and not tonsillectomy.

2.11 ACE

Wilms' nephroblastoma is the most common of all childhood malignant tumours accounting for 10% of cases. It presents before 5 years of age in 80% of children (median age of 3.5 years), 95% are unilateral and 20% have metastasised at presentation, mainly to the lung and liver. Eighty per cent present with an abdominal mass, 25% with haematuria and approximately 30% with flank pain. Other features include failure to thrive and hemihypertrophy. Wilms' may be sporadic or familial, in which case it may be associated with aniridia, genito-urinary malformations and retardation (WAGR syndrome). The Wilms' tumour gene is found on chromosome 11.

Investigations of choice include intravenous urethrogram (renal pelvis distortion, hydronephrosis), USS and CT. Renal biopsy should be avoided. Treatment involves nephrectomy, chemotherapy (eg actinomycin E) and radiotherapy which can be curative (80% 5-year survival).

2.12 CE

Undescended testis occurs in 2–3% of term male neonates but in 15–30% of premature babies. Only 25% of cases are bilateral. If the testis is truly undescended it will lie anywhere along the path of descent from the abdominal cavity. Other sites include the perineum, femoral region or base of penis. Orchidopexy must be performed before 2 years of age to preserve function, preferably at 1 year. There is an increased incidence of torsion and also neoplasia (eg seminoma) which persists despite surgery.

2.13 ADE

Common side-effects of sodium valproate include gastric irritation, nausea, ataxia and tremor, hyperammonaemia, increased appetite and weight gain, and transient hair loss (regrowth may be curly) – also impaired liver function and rarely pancreatitis. Stevens–Johnson syndrome is a typical side-effect of phenytoin and hyperactivity is usually associated with clonazepam and phenobarbitone, sodium valproate being more commonly linked with drowsiness.

2.14 ABCDE

Infection with the parainfluenza viruses and rhinovirus is particularly likely to precipitate an acute asthma attack.

2.15 CE

High-risk infants do not require skin testing before vaccination up to 3 months of age. The BCG should only be given after a negative tuberculin test. BCG may be given with other live vaccines, otherwise a gap of more than 3 weeks should be observed between injections or a suboptimal response to both vaccines may ensue. Live oral polio vaccine (OPV), which works by inducing gut immunity, is the exception and can be given at any time. HIV infection is an absolute contraindication to BCG vaccination.

2.16 BE

The fetus is most at risk in the first 16 weeks of gestation, with approximately 55% affected if maternal infection occurs in the first 4 weeks. Cataract is associated with infection at 8–9 weeks, deafness at 5–7 weeks (although it may occur with second trimester infection) and cardiac lesions at 5–10 weeks. Other features include purpura, jaundice, hepatosplenomegaly, microcephaly, microphthalmia, retinopathy, developmental delay, cerebral palsy and thrombocytopenia. Miscarriage or stillbirth may also occur.

2.17 BC

The 'incidence' is the number of new cases occurring during a specified period in a defined population, whereas the 'prevalence' is the number of cases at any particular time or during a specified period of time in a defined population. Therefore an acute illness will have a high incidence, but low prevalence, whereas the annual incidence of a chronic illness will be much lower than its prevalence. Both are expressed as a rate per 1000 of the population. The NMR is the number of deaths of live born babies up to 1 month of age per 1000 live births and the IMR is the number of deaths of all infants under 1 year of age per 1000 live births.

2.18 AD

Apgar scores are usually recorded at 1 minute, 5 minutes and at 5-minute intervals after birth.

Score	Pulse	Respiratory rate	Muscle tone	Reflex on suction	Colour
0	0	Nil	Limp	Nil	White
1	< 100	Slow/irregular	Limp/flexion	Grimace	Blue
2	> 100	Regular	Active	Cough	Pink

Table 2 The parameters for Apgar scores

2.19 ABDE

Depression may often initially present with various psychosomatic symptoms (eg abdominal pain, headache). However, the presence of an actual chronic physical disease (eg asthma, diabetes) is a predisposing factor and various medications, including steroids and some anticonvulsants, can also result in depression. Depression may also present with behavioural problems such as vandalism or drug abuse and younger children may regress, resulting in, for example, secondary enuresis.

2.20 BDE

At birth, 1% of hips are found to be unstable and are more common on the left (60%) with one in five being bilateral. Risk factors include female sex (80%), family history, breech delivery, first child and history of oligohydramnios. Screening involves the Ortolani–Barlow manoeuvre with USS of suspicious joints, which shows the shape of the cartilaginous socket and position of the femoral head (X-rays are unhelpful before 6 weeks). If these tests are positive, neonates should be splinted in abduction for 6–12 weeks with clinical and radiological follow-up at 3, 6 and 12 months. Most hips will have stabilised with conservative methods; however, persistent instability will need surgery. This is more likely if initial treatment was delayed.

2.21 ABCDE

A prolonged neonatal jaundice due to conjugated hyperbilirubinaemia is a known presenting feature of cystic fibrosis and should be investigated. However, a sweat test may be difficult to do in neonates, so alternative tests may be necessary (eg immune reactive trypsin). Any child with failure to thrive or short stature, especially if associated with respiratory or gastro-intestinal symptoms, should also be investigated for cystic fibrosis. Pancreatic enzyme and dietary supplements are needed and may have to be increased when the child is ill (overnight tube feeding may be of benefit). Chest infections are common and cause progressive lung damage (ie bronchiectasis). The usual pathogens isolated are *Haemophilus influenzae*, *S. aureus*, *Klebsiella* and *Pseudomonas*. Treatment includes chest physiotherapy, iv antibiotics and nebulised bronchodilators.

2.22 BC

Roseola infantum is a common disease of infancy. It is commonly due to human herpes virus type 6 (herpes virus type 7 is also a likely pathogen). It has an incubation period of approximately 5–15 days, then typically presents with a high fever for 3–4 days which subsides as a fine maculopapular rash that develops initially on the torso before becoming widespread. It resolves in 2–3 days.

Human parvovirus type B19 is the cause of the 'fifth disease', which is also known as the 'slapped cheek' syndrome and erythema infectiosum. Roseola infantum is also known as the 'sixth disease' and its only significant complication is febrile convulsions. Measles and chickenpox are associated with pneumonia.

2.23 ABC

Homocystinuria is a metabolic disorder associated with tall stature. Endocrine disorders resulting in tall stature include hyperthyroidism, precocious puberty and growth hormone excess (pituitary gigantism). Endocrine disorders resulting in short stature include pseudohypoparathyroidism, growth hormone deficiency, hypopituitarism, hypothyroidism and Cushing's syndrome.

2.24 CDE

Cromoglycate is ineffective in the treatment of acute asthma but is a useful prophylactic agent. Inhalers deliver less than 5% of the drug to the lungs and even nebulisers only deliver less than 10%. Aminophylline can be used in the management of an acute attack, however the loading dose should be omitted if the child is already on oral theophylline and ideally the drug level should be measured before the infusion is commenced. Regular low-dose inhaled steroids do not result in growth retardation. The incidence of oral candidiasis can be reduced if steroids are inhaled via a spacer device and rinsing the mouth afterwards reduces the risk further.

2.25 BCE

Primary prevention is aimed at preventing the 'accident' from happening and includes speed limits, stair gates, teaching road safety and child-proof catches on cupboards. Secondary prevention aims to prevent injury should the 'accident' happen. Examples of secondary prevention include cycling helmets, seat belts, smoke alarms and fire extinguishers kept in the house. NB Child-resistant lids are a form of primary prevention as they prevent the child from reaching the drug; however, blister packs for prescription drugs merely limit the number of a tablets a child can get at in a given time and are therefore a form of secondary prevention. Tertiary prevention aims to limit the impact of an injury once the 'accident' has happened and includes teaching parents first aid skills and providing good access to the emergency services.

2.26 ABE

The Dubowitz system is a system for estimating the gestational age of neonates from 26 to 44 weeks. It includes various neurological criteria (eg posture, head lag) and physical (or external) criteria which include: presence of oedema; skin texture; skin colour (not crying); skin opacity (trunk); lanugo (over back); plantar creases; nipple formation; breast size; ear form and firmness; and development of genitalia (ie presence of testes in scrotum).

2.27 ABC

Infants born to poorly controlled diabetic mothers may have sacral agenesis, hypomagnesaemia, hypocalcaemia, polycythaemia and Erb's palsy secondary to the increased risk of shoulder dystocia.

2.28 CE

Trimethoprim is usually the best first-line antibiotic, as *E. coli* (responsible for 80% of UTIs) is often resistant to amoxicillin. Augmentin, nitrofurantoin and cephalosporins are also useful. Trimethoprim and nitrofurantoin are often used for prophylaxis in children with vesico-ureteric reflux (VUR), and are effective when given once daily. Prevention of UTIs includes the avoidance of constipation, ensuring the bladder is completely empty after voiding and wiping in a front-to-back direction. If there is no evidence of chronic pyelonephritis then treatment of asymptomatic bacteriuria is not recommended as it may allow a virulent strain to re-infect with the elimination of an avirulent one. Surgery may be necessary if the UTI is secondary to calculi, obstruction or severe VUR.

2.29 BE

Cerebral palsy is a disorder of posture and movement resulting from a non-progressive lesion of the developing brain before or during the neonatal period. The expression of the lesion changes as the brain matures. It has a prevalence of 2.5 in 1000. Mental handicap occurs in < 50% of children. Other associated disabilities include visual (25%), language (90%) and hearing loss (25%). The importance of the various causes of cerebral palsy is controversial. Perinatal insult is now thought to be less important as an aetiological factor. Other causes include cryptogenic (35%), genetic (20%), postnatal disease, eg meningitis (20%) and intra-uterine infection, irradiation or drug-induced damage (5%). Diagnosis of cerebral palsy under 6 months may be difficult unless it is severe. Similarly, mild cases may only present with delayed developmental milestones or clumsiness.

2.30 A

The stepwise treatment of asthma involves starting at the 'step' most appropriate for the severity and moving up or down as needed. Treatment can be gradually 'stepped down' if control has been good for over 6 months.

Step 1: try occasional β-agonists – if required more than daily then treatment should progress to include the steps 2–5

Step 2: inhaled cromoglycate, nedocromil or low-dose inhaled steroids

Step 3: high-dose inhaled steroids or low-dose inhaled steroids plus long-acting inhaled β-agonist

Step 4: high-dose inhaled steroids plus trials of inhaled long-acting β-agonists, theophylline, ipratropium bromide, oral long-acting β-agonists

Step 5: addition of regular oral steroids

2.31 A

Asthma affects > 10% of children and causes approximately 50 deaths per year in the UK. Most are teenagers with chronic severe asthma. The prevalence has been gradually increasing over the past 20 years. This may be due to increased parental awareness, pollution and changing infant feeding patterns. The mortality has, however, remained static.

2.32 ABE

The gene for cystic fibrosis is located on the long arm of chromosome 7 and analysis of fetal DNA obtained in the first trimester (at chorionic villous biopsy) will confirm the diagnosis. The gene carrier rate is 1 in 22 of the Caucasian population and approximately 75–80% of these gene mutations in the UK are due to a deletion at delta F508, although this frequency varies geographically (eg in Italy, it is only responsible for about 40% of mutations). Cystic fibrosis is an autosomal recessive disorder, therefore two carrier parents have a 1 in 2 chance of having a carrier child, a 1 in 4 chance of having a normal child and a 1 in 4 chance of having an affected child.

2.33 AC

Generalised 'absences' present between 3 and 13 years and are more common in girls. 'Absences' characteristically last less than 10 seconds and recur more than 10 times a day. There is no collapse and the patient is usually unaware of them. Affected children have a normal IQ but may have learning difficulties secondary to the frequency of the attacks. The EEG shows a bilateral symmetrical 3 Hz spike and wave pattern, which may be precipitated by hyperventilation (EEG spike waves over Rolandic are typical of simple partial seizures). A CT scan reveals no structural abnormality and the cause is unknown, though they may have a familial predisposition. It usually remits in adult life, but 30% go on to develop generalised tonic-clonic epilepsy. First-line treatment is with valproate or ethosuximide.

2.34 ACD

Constipation is the passage of hard, dry stools resulting in distress for the child. However, it may present as diarrhoea when constipation with overflow is present. Breast-fed babies may pass infrequent soft stools (eg weekly), but this is a normal variation and parents should be reassured. Constipation is most commonly secondary to a low-fibre diet and other causes include anal fissures, medication, dehydration, anal trauma (eg post-operative, abuse) and spinal disorders (eg spina bifida). Mental disability is associated with failure to develop a regular bowel habit, however Down's syndrome is also associated with an increased incidence of Hirschsprung's disease.

2.35 CDE

The Butler-Schloss report recommends that parents should be invited to attend all or part of the conference, unless the chairperson feels their presence will be detrimental to the child's interests. Ideally a case conference should be held with parental consent/involvement without an EPO being necessary. However, if an EPO is necessary then this may be a convenient time to have the conference. A senior officer from social services must act as the chairperson. Other invitees include the GP, paediatrician, police child protection team, a solicitor from the local authority and other specialists as appropriate. The case conference acts in an advisory capacity only and considers the evidence of abuse, the cause, the risk of recurrence and safety of any siblings. However, apart from deciding whether to put the child on the Child Protection Register, all other decisions are made by the directors of social services, who will obviously take into consideration the findings of the case conference.

2.36 ACD

Reye's syndrome is acute encephalopathy with fatty degeneration of the liver, kidneys and pancreas, resulting in vomiting, delirium, fits and coma. Other features include hepatomegaly, hypoglycaemia, cerebral oedema and hyperammonaemia. The aetiology is unclear, but viral illness and aspirin exposure have been postulated as precipitating risk factors. Indeed there has been a steady decline in incidence since 1986 when aspirin was withdrawn from use in young children. It usually presents before the age of 2 years after a prodromal illness and is associated with a high mortality. The transaminases are typically elevated, but bilirubin is usually normal. Treatment involves general supportive measures and reduction of any raised intracranial pressures with normalisation of the $PaCO_2$ and iv mannitol. Complications include renal failure, gastro-intestinal bleeding and pancreatitis and should be managed accordingly.

2.37 CE

The characteristic features of Fallot's tetralogy are a ventricular septal defect (VSD), pulmonary stenosis, an overriding aorta and ventricular hypertrophy resulting in a right-to-left shunt. Fallot's tetralogy and TGA are the two leading causes of cyanotic congenital heart disease. In Fallot's tetralogy central cyanosis occurs with infundibular spasm which is relieved by propranolol. There is no murmur associated with the VSD; however, the pulmonary stenosis typically results in an ejection systolic murmur heard best over the pulmonary area. The characteristic chest X-ray appearance of Fallot's tetralogy is a 'boot shaped' cardiac shadow, whereas the 'egg on its side' is more typical of TGA.

2.38 A

Vasoconstriction of the ophthalmic artery occurs in simple migraine resulting in transient visual aura, scintillating scotoma, zigzag lines (fortification phenomenon), visual field defects and micropsia. Strabismus, diplopia and nystagmus are all signs of possible intracranial pathology. Papilloedema is a sign of raised intracranial pressure indicating more serious intracranial pathology.

2.39 ABC

Down's syndrome is the leading cause of severe learning difficulties. It affects approximately 1 in 660 births. Trisomy 21 is responsible for 90% of cases and has a recurrence risk of about 1%. The incidence increases with maternal age, with woman of 40 years having a 1 in 40 risk. Typical features include developmental delay with an IQ between 20 and 75. They have a characteristic appearance of up-slanting eyes with wide epicanthic folds, a small nose with a low bridge, a small mouth with a protruding tongue, a single palmar crease and general hypotonia/ joint laxity. A cardiac lesion, particularly a patent ductus arteriosus (PDA) or atrial septal defect (ASD), is present in 40%. Other common disorders include duodenal atresia, thyroid disease and leukaemia.

2.40 BCDE

Both haemophilia A and B are X-linked disorders and result from deficient factor VIII coagulation. In both conditions the intrinsic clotting pathway is affected resulting in a prolonged activated thromboplastin ratio (APTR). The prothrombin time measures the extrinsic pathway and is therefore normal. Haemophilia presents with an increased risk of haemorrhage, resulting in bruising, recurrent haemarthroses (leading to progressive joint destruction) and following surgery or dental extraction rendering prophylactic dental care essential. Management of acute bleeds requires the prompt administration of factor VIII concentrate (or cryoprecipitate/FFP). Patients must never receive aspirin or be given intramuscular injections and a haematological opinion should be sought prior to any surgical procedure.

2.41 AB

In the UK, cows' milk protein intolerance is the most common cause of chronic diarrhoea in infants under 1 year of age. Other common causes include constipation with overflow, post gastroenteritis (eg lactose intolerance), infections (eg *Salmonella*, *Giardia*) and toddler diarrhoea which is suggested by recognisable food in the stool, is of unknown cause and is not of any sinister significance. Coeliac disease is due to sensitivity to gluten in wheat and rye, which causes the characteristic jejunal villous atrophy seen at biopsy and leads to malabsorption. However, this is not diagnostic, as similar appearances may be found with gastroenteritis and cows' milk intolerance. Diagnosis is confirmed by clinical remission within weeks of commencing a gluten-free diet and associated reduction in the number of circulating IgA-specific antibodies. It has an incidence of about 1 in 2000 and tends to run in families with girls being more commonly affected. It usually presents at between 9 months and 3 years with failure to thrive and frequent loose stools, although mild cases may remain undiagnosed into adulthood. Diffuse inflammation and ulceration of the colon characterise ulcerative colitis; it is rare in childhood and is not inherited in a mendelian fashion.

2.42 ABDE

Appendicitis is rare in the under-fives, but nearly 90% of cases present with perforation demonstrating the difficulty in diagnosis. Problems may be due to the child's ineloquent history and because of its rarity it is not considered initially. In addition it may be difficult to localise pain in a small abdomen. Retrocaecal appendicitis may not cause any localising signs (PR reveals tenderness anteriorly) or the child may present with urinary symptoms/signs if a pelvic appendix is inflamed. A useful sign is the child's ability to 'hop' or 'jump' as peritonitis is excluded if this is painless, making the diagnosis of appendicitis unlikely. Differential diagnoses include mesenteric adenitis, UTI, diabetic ketoacidosis, intussusception, lower lobe pneumonia and infectious hepatitis.

2.43 AB

The health visitor relieves the midwife of responsibility at 10 days post delivery and is subsequently responsible for child health surveillance in all children up to 5 years of age. They are informed of every child under 5 who attends A&E and are then obliged to contact the health visitor of any child who needs appropriate follow-up. They also supervise the running of immunisation clinics; however, social workers are responsible for children in care.

2.44 ABE

Anorexia nervosa occurs predominantly amongst teenage girls, affecting 1 in 250 between the ages of 15 and 18 years, although boys represent up to 5% of cases. Features include persistent refusal to eat leading to potentially dangerous weight loss, intense fear of becoming obese, disturbed perception of body image and primary or secondary amenorrhoea due to endocrine disturbance (low luteinising hormone (LH), follicle stimulating hormone (FSH) and oestrogen). NB Amenorrhoea before weight loss should arouse suspicion of hypothalamic dysfunction.

Symptoms may include excessive exercise, laxative/diuretic abuse and induction of vomiting which may result in hypokalaemia. Other physical complications include sensitivity to cold, constipation, faints, lethargy, hypotension and hypoglycaemia. The aetiology is multifactorial with family dynamics a key issue. Management involves gaining the patient's trust and outpatient psychotherapy for mild cases. Admission in severe cases involves treatment of medical complications, family therapy, individual psychotherapy including privileges for weight gain and occasionally drugs (eg anxiolytics, antidepressants). Depression and suicide attempts are common. Approximately 50% remain underweight with psychological difficulties and the overall mortality rates are up to 8%.

2.45 CDE

Neisseria gonorrhoeae may cause ophthalmia neonatorum, however *Chlamydia* is more frequently responsible. Stevens–Johnson syndrome is a systemic disorder associated with erythema multiforme ('target' lesions), fever, mouth, genital and eye ulcers. Orbital cellulitis presents with significant orbital oedema, limitation of ocular movements, fever, and altered colour vision as a late feature. Causes include adjacent sinusitis, bacteraemia and other local infection. Intrauterine infections which predispose to neonatal cataracts include toxoplasmosis, rubella, cytomegalovirus (CMV), herpes simplex and varicella. Other causes include autosomal inheritance and chromosomal disorders (eg Down's syndrome), metabolic disorders (eg diabetes mellitus), trauma and the use of systemic steroids. Glaucoma is rare in childhood and results from defective drainage of aqueous humour from the anterior chamber. It may be due to primary causes such as aniridia or secondary causes such as iritis, trauma or intraocular tumour.

Answers to Extended Matching Questions

2.46 Choice of investigations

1 H – Haemoglobin electrophoresis

The most likely cause of dactylitis in a 6-month-old child is sickle cell disease. The investigation that would diagnose this is Hb electrophoresis.

2 B – Bone marrow aspiration cytology

The most likely cause for this is immune thrombocytopenic purpura (ITP), however aplastic anaemia is possible, as is ALL. Bone marrow aspiration cytology is the investigation that would give a definitive diagnosis.

3 I – Monospot

A 14-year-old boy with this history is most likely to have glandular fever, a monospot would definitively diagnose this.

2.47 Decisions about life-saving treatment

1 B – The 'no chance' situation

2 E – The 'unbearable' situation

3 C – The 'no purpose' situation

The RCPCH issued guidelines in 1997 on when it could be considered appropriate to 'withdraw or withhold lifesaving treatment'. The five situations are:

- The brain-dead child – when the formal criteria for brain-death are met.
- The persistent vegetative state (PVS) – when the formal criteria for PVS are met.
- The 'no chance' situation – where, despite all treatments there is no chance of the child surviving, it could be considered that withdrawal of care is appropriate.

- The 'no purpose' situation – where a child may survive given the necessary interventions but they will be so impaired that they will probably not achieve 'personhood' and be able to make decisions about their own life.
- The 'unbearable' situation – where the treatment is so invasive and has so many side-effects that it may be more than the child can bear (the treatment is worse than the disease).

It is important to note that withdrawing and withholding treatment from children should be done as part of a multi-disciplinary process with full parental involvement.

2.48 Heart defects

1 E – Innocent (flow) murmur

This is an incidental finding in a presumably acyanotic, otherwise healthy 3-year-old. The murmur is soft, ejection systolic at the LSE only and so a flow murmur is the most likely diagnosis (due to the increased flow as the child is unwell). The GP should re-examine once this acute illness has resolved.

2 F – PDA

This is not a cyanotic lesion. As she is only 12 hours old then the most likely diagnosis is a PDA that has yet to close. Full femoral pulses are usually felt in PDA.

3 B – ASD

Again an acyanotic lesion. The murmur heard is a pulmonary flow murmur due to the increased flow. The flow through the defect itself is not great enough (as atrial) to produce a murmur. A fixed split of the second heart sound is classic of an ASD. Hepatomegaly is a characteristic sign of heart failure in infants and small children.

2.49 Common infections

1 D – Epstein–Barr virus

Glandular fever should always be considered in older children with sore throats. Amoxicillin if given when a child has EBV infection will cause a florid macular-papular rash. This is one way of making the diagnosis!

2 C – Coxsackie virus A16

Vesicles on the hands and feet, and probably in the mouth if refusing food, is why hand, foot and mouth disease has that name. It is caused by Coxsackie A16 and it is very contagious. Nurseries often close while there is an outbreak.

3 F – *Mycoplasma pneumoniae*

Target lesions are seen in erythema multiforme (EM). In an unwell child with EM *Mycoplasma* infection should always be considered, as must herpes simplex infection. Stevens–Johnson syndrome is an important complication.

2.50 Statistics and research methods

1 C – Lead time

2 E – Likelihood ratio

3 J – Specificity

- Lead time: the time between a condition being identified by screening and when it would become clinically apparent.
- Lag time: the time between an intervention being assessed as clinically useful and when it actually enters every day practice.
- Sensitivity: percentage of those, who have a condition, who are correctly tested positive.
- Specificity: percentage of those, who do not have a condition, who are correctly tested negative.

- Likelihood ratio: odds of a positive test result in an affected individual compared with that of a positive result in an unaffected individual – this is a positive likelihood ratio.
- Number needed to treat: the number of patients who would need to have an intervention for a set outcome to be shown in one of them.
- Prevalence: the total number of cases in a population at any one time (expressed as a proportion of the total population).
- Incidence: rate at which new cases of a condition occur in a population (over a set period of time – usually 1 year).

2.51 Immediate interventions

1 J – Vagal manoeuvres

Any child in SVT should have vagal manoeuvres tried first as they are quick and easy (and can be effective). The strategies that can be used are: an older child can try a Valsalva manoeuvre by blowing up a balloon. Infants can have their face immersed in cold water to try to elicit a diving reflex. Unilateral carotid massage can also be tried.

2 I – Synchronous DC shock – 0.5 J/kg

The low saturations and prolonged capillary refill indicate that the child is in shock. A shocked child in VT but with a pulse should undergo asynchronous DC cardioversion at an initial power of 0.5 J/kg (should be performed following rapid sequence induction anaesthesia). The underlying diagnosis is a likely tricyclic-antidepressant overdose.

3 D – Asynchronous DC Shock – 2 J/kg

Treatment of VF/pulseless VT is with asynchronous DC shock of 2 J/kg (followed by a further 2 J/kg, then 4 J/kg). Cardio-pulmonary resuscitation (CPR) must continue when the shocks are not being given, and it is important to give adrenaline (epinephrine) – but only DC shock will convert the rhythm to sinus.

All these answers are taken from the *Advanced Paediatric Life Support – The Practical Approach*, 3rd edition, 2001. BMJ Books.

2.52 Neoplasms

1 B – Acute lymphoblastic leukaemia

Acute lymphoblastic leukaemia is the most common malignancy in childhood (35–40% of all childhood malignancies). The incidence is highest in early childhood. Diagnosis is made on bone marrow aspiration; however, blast cells can often be seen in the peripheral blood. The treatment generally lasts for around 2 years. Survival rates are as high as 85% at 5 years.

2 J – Wilms' tumour

There are only two likely diagnoses in this case – Wilms' nephroblastoma or neuroblastoma. As there is blood in the urine then there is probably renal involvement and therefore a Wilms' is the more likely of the two.

For further details see question 2.11 (page 131). Both Wilms' and neuroblastomas count for 8% each of all childhood malignancies.

3 G – Non-Hodgkin's lymphoma

This is a typical history for non-Hodgkin's lymphoma. The shortness of breath is due to mediastinal involvement (which can ultimately cause superior vena cava (SVC) obstruction). The staging and treatment of non-Hodgkin's lymphoma are essentially the same as in adults. Lymphomas count for 15% of all childhood malignancies and are the second most common solid tumours after the central nervous system (CNS) tumours. The other childhood malignancies are bone tumours (7%), retinoblastoma (2%), and others such as rhabdomyosarcoma or adenocarcinoma.

2.53 Gastro-intestinal disorders

1 D – Crohn's disease

From the history, and the objective weight loss, there is likely to be a significant pathology ongoing. The time course is a little lengthy to be infective, although not impossible. The inflammatory markers are raised, indicating an ongoing inflammatory process. The perianal skin tags should strongly raise the suspicion of Crohn's disease. This disease is increasing in childhood and the current incidence is between 10 and 25 per 100, 000. It is an inflammatory process involving the whole bowel (mouth to anus). Clinically patients present with abdominal pain, weight loss/reduced growth and diarrhoea. On examination there may mouth ulceration, and perianal lesions. Extragastro-intestinal features may be present – including arthralgia, anaemia and uveitis. Radiological contrast studies will show involvement of various parts of the bowel (skip lesions), There may also be signs of inflammation –'cobblestones' or 'rose-thorn' ulcers. Treatment should be shared with a tertiary level, multidisciplinary, paediatric gastro-enterological team.

2 H – Toddler's diarrhoea

This is a classic history for toddler's diarrhoea. The child is well and thriving but the parents can understandably be anxious. The cause is thought to be due a fast enteric transit time, and a brisk gastrocolic reflex. Reassurance is vital, but simple measures such as reducing fruit juice intake may help.

3 J – Viral gastro-enteritis

This is an acute history so an infective process is likely; the fact that her sibling had a similar illness again makes an infective cause much more likely. A viral cause is more common in this age group (eg rotavirus). Viral gastro-enteritis is a self-limiting condition but there is a risk of dehydration if oral intake is insufficient. Medications such as loperamide or codeine to 'reduce' the diarrhoea have no place in management, and may lengthen the duration of the illness. Secondary lactose intolerance is uncommon and before changing the milk to a lactose-free formula, stool reducing sugars should be checked.

2.54

1 I – Small genetic height potential

This child may not have a big genetic height potential (ie her overall potential height that she will get from her genetic make-up) if both her parents are not tall. It is unlikely that she will be tall.

2 C – Constitutional delay in growth and puberty

There are no clinical signs of puberty yet in this boy except that his testicular volume is 8 ml. The pubertal growth spurt normally starts once the testicular volume reaches 10 ml. The delayed bone age means that there is still growth potential in the bones so that if the bone age is delayed 2 years then once puberty starts he will have an 'extra' 2 years of growth compared to his peers. Constitutional delay of growth and puberty can be managed with reassurance, however peer pressure and bullying at school may lead some families to want intervention. In these cases a short course of testosterone may 'kick start' the growth.

3 F – Hypothyroidism

The features of constipation, weight gain and academic faltering are consistent with hypothyroidism. Acquired hypothyroidism is due to two main causes: autoimmune (Hashimoto's) thyroiditis and post-total-body irradiation (TBI). Worldwide the most common cause is iodine deficiency. Since part of the preparation for bone marrow transplant requires TBI this is the most likely cause. Treatment is with thyroxine replacement.

Best of Five Answers

2.55 C: Anywhere on the body, as long as only the hand is used and no mark is left

This is the law as it stands at present. The hand must be open (not a clenched fist), no implement may be used and 'no injury' inflicted (so it must leave no mark). It could well be argued that even if no mark is left, an 'injury' may still have been inflicted.

2.56 B: Seven-day trial of lactulose (10 ml bd)

Dietary advice is always an integral part of the management of constipation. A diet with adequate fibre, fruit and vegetable and fluid intake should be encouraged. However, in this case some lactulose will help soften the stools to allow a normal bowel habit to be re-established. Senna would also achieve this but can cause stomach cramps and less compliance.

2.57 C: He must not be circumcised

While all of the pieces of advice are valid – it is most important to advise that circumcision should not take place. Many parents are keen for circumcision for ethnic or religious reasons; however, circumcision can make a surgical hypospadias repair much more difficult.

2.58 B: Blood film

Some of these investigations are more useful than others. An abdominal USS will detect the enlargement of abdominal/para-aortic lymph nodes but not help in establishing a diagnosis. A Paul Bunnell test, if positive, will establish a diagnosis, but this is unlikely given the history. CRP/LFTs and amylase may indicate an inflammatory process but again will not help establish a diagnosis. A blood film would be the most useful given the history (leukaemia, haematopoietic disorders).

2.59 E: Regular antipyretics and analgesics with review in 48 hours

Antibiotics are of limited benefit in the treatment of otitis media. They can shorten the duration of the illness but the number needed to treat is 17. Eighty per cent of the cases of otitis media resolve without treatment. Supportive measures such as antipyretics and analgesics are important measures to recommend to parents. Glasziou, P.P., Del Mar, C.B., Sanders, S.L. and Hayem M. 2003. Antibiotics for acute otitis media in children (Cochrane Review). *In: Cochrane Library, Issue 4.*

2.60 D: Intraventricular haemorrhage

The initial cranial USS in a 25/40 gestation infant is primarily to look for intraventricular haemorrhage since the period in which it is most likely to happen is the initial 48 hours. The other features are important but may well not be seen initially.

2.61 A: Direct and indirect bilirubin

All of these are important elements of a prolonged jaundice screen. Biliary atresia is the important cause of conjugated hyperbilirubinaemia. It is surgically corrected by the Kasai procedure and this should be done before 60 days (8 weeks) of life otherwise the outcome is markedly worse. TFTs are theoretically not so important to perform as the Guthrie test should screen for hypothyroidism. The other tests are not as urgent as the split bilirubin.

2.62 C: Admit for enteral rehydration via a nasogastric tube

Enteral rehydration using an oral rehydration solution is almost invariably the preferred way of rehydrating children. If a child is not tolerating small frequent feeds then nasogastric rehydration is an underused next best step. The fluid can be run through a continuous pump so that it is better tolerated. IV fluids are effective but can have profound effects on the serum electrolyte balance if not monitored closely. Most children will tolerate fluids in an emergency department, but failure to take fluids orally is not an indication for iv therapy.

2.63 C: Hepatitis B vaccine and hepatitis B immunoglobulin

Hepatitis B sAb +ve, eAg +ve is classified as high risk of infectivity to the infant. The babies in such cases should receive both the hepatitis B vaccine and hepatitis B immunoglobulin within the first 24 hours of life. Low-risk infants (sAb +ve, eAg –ve) should receive hepatitis vaccine only.

2.64 C: Wave bye-bye

Brush teeth with help: by 26 months

Play ball with examiner: by 17 months

Wave bye-bye: by 15 months

Put on a T-shirt unaided: by 3 years

Play 'pat-a-cake': by 11 months

See neurodevelopmental milestones (page 214)

2.65 B: Star chart

A star chart for dry nights is a useful tool for managing nocturnal enuresis. Simple measures such as minimising fluid intake before bed and ensuring the child goes to the loo before going to bed are important. Medical interventions are not a good first-line measure – desmopressin is effective but there is a high relapse rate off treatment. Imipramine is infrequently used now since there are more effective treatments and it has serious side-effects. Enuresis clinics provide good support but the majority do not accept referrals for children under 7 years old.

2.66 C: Hop on one leg

Able to run steadily: by 20 months

Walk backwards: by 16 months

Hop on one leg: by 4 years

Walk up stairs unaided: by 20 months

Throw ball overhand: 3 years

See neurodevelopmental milestones (page 214)

2.67 A: Police protection order

If the child is thought to be in immediate danger then a PPO is the quickest and most effective as it allows the child to be taken to a place of safety. An EPO Court Wardship and temporary fostering may occur later but not immediately. A section 47 meeting is convened by social services for professionals and family to assess a child's needs and the ability of the current carer to ensure a safe and nurturing environment.

2.68 E: Femoral nerve block

Femoral nerve block is a safe and very effective method of pain relief for limb injuries. The other options are, of course, useful but probably not sufficiently strong for this severity of injury. Splinting is vital but analgesia should be given first. IV morphine should be used with caution if there is the possibility of a significant head injury (APLS 3rd edition).

2.69 A: Tuberous sclerosis

Tuberous sclerosis – autosomal dominant, 1 in 50, 000.

- 'Ash leaf' macules (from infancy) – depigmented lesions approximately 1–2 cm long
- 'Shagreen' patches – (from 2 years) areas of roughened skin, usually sacral, likened to shark skin
- Adenoma sebaceum – (from 5 years) – 1- to 2-mm papules usually facial (butterfly distribution)
- Epilepsy (usually before 2 years)

Neurofibromatosis type 1 – autosomal dominant, 1 in 2500.

- Café-au-lait spots (> 2 in children under 5 years, > 5 in children over 5 years is significant)
- Axillary freckling
- Neurofibromata (from 12 years) – papules anywhere on the body
- Epilepsy only in 10%

Ataxia telangiectasia – autosomal recessive, a chromosomal repair defect. Affected childred present as late walkers. Ataxia develops in early childhood and is progressive.

- Conjunctival telangiectasia develop from 5 years

Incontinentia pigmenti – X-linked dominant.

- Vesicular stage – neonatal period, linear distribution; resolves by 1 month
- Verrucose stage – 1–4 months, warty lesions appearing mainly on limbs; resolves by 6 months
- Whorl stage – by 2 years, linear and whorl pattern of hyperpigmentation on limbs
- Epilepsy in over 30%

Sturge–Weber – sporadic, 1 in 50, 000.

- Naevus in trigeminal distribution with an ipsilateral leptomeningeal haemangioma
- Intracranial calcification is common, especially in the occipital region
- Seizures develop in early childhood

2.70 A: Minimal change disease

Minimal change disease is by far the most common cause of nephrotic syndrome in childhood. The next most common is focal segmental glomerular sclerosis. Finnish microcystic disease is a rare cause of nephrotic syndrome seen only in infancy.

2.71 D: Left basal chest infection

The history and site of the pain are unlikely for appendicitis, mesenteric adenitis and pyelonephritis. A UTI is unlikely with no symptoms and a negative dipstick. A basal pneumonia is an important differential diagnosis in a febrile child who presents with abdominal pain.

2.72 B: Trial of Gaviscon

This is a difficult situation and different practitioners may have different views. If there is a clear history for GOR then a trial of Gaviscon is simple and has minimal side-effects and is therefore a reasonable approach. If there is an improvement in the symptoms further treatment can be initiated as warranted. There is an argument that since the child is thriving the GOR is something the child will outgrow, but is an indication for treatment in the interim. A pH study or barium swallow is a good investigation for diagnosing severity of GOR; however, if there are good clinical features this may be academic.

2.73 A: Administer activated charcoal and take paracetamol levels at 4 hours

Five pills is not a toxic dose. Since the overdose was within 1 hour activated charcoal may reduce systemic absorption and is worth giving (if she will take it!). Levels for paracetamol and salicylate should be taken at 4 hours to assess whether treatment is needed (as she may have concealed what and how much she actually took). All overdoses should, ideally, be discussed with the National Poisons Information Service (NPIS), especially if staggered overdose or more than one substance was taken. Most A&E Departments now have online access to 'Toxbase' – the NPIS website that allows quick referencing for overdose management.

2.74 C: Admit her for formal assessment by a child psychiatrist

Any child who has taken a deliberate overdose, even if no medical treatment is required, must be seen by a child psychiatrist. These children must not be discharged until assessed safe to do so from a psychiatrist. This means that the majority will be admitted until assessed, though some may be seen in A&E depending on the level of psychiatric service provided.

PAPER 3 ANSWERS

Multiple Choice Answers

3.1 BE

Glue ear causes a conductive hearing loss and the resulting deafness may present with behavioural problems due to the child's frustration. The natural history of the condition means that most children will have normal hearing by 8 years of age regardless. However, early treatment is vital to ensure that the hearing is adequate for normal development. Surgical treatment involves myringotomy and insertion of grommets; the latter allows the middle ear to be ventilated – a role that will eventually be resumed by the eustachian tube. The majority are extruded 2 months to 2 years following insertion.

3.2 AE

Hib infection is rare before 3 months, the incidence then steadily rises peaking at approximately 10–11 months and then declining to the age of 4 years. All children less than 13 months should therefore receive the full vaccination course. From 13 months to 2 years unimmunised children should receive a single Hib dose with their MMR (children are less at risk in this age group and therefore a single dose is effective). The Hib vaccine is not live and is therefore safe in immunocompromised patients. Sixty per cent of invasive Hib disease presents as meningitis, 15% presents as epiglottitis, 10% presents as septicaemia alone and the remaining 15% includes septic arthritis, osteomyelitis, cellulitis, pneumonia and pericarditis. It has a mortality rate of approximately 2%.

3.3 ABCDE

Health promotion is now a major part of health policy in 'Health of the Nation' targets for ischaemic heart disease and stroke, mental illness, HIV and sexual health, cancer and accident prevention. Important areas relating specifically to children and adolescents include smoking, alcohol consumption, illegal substance abuse, healthy diets, obesity, suicide, deliberate self-harm, accidents, teenage pregnancy and sexually transmitted disease.

3.4 BE

Between 0 and 1 year an infant should ideally have at least five recordings of weight and probably one or two recordings of length; between 1 and 2 years they should have at least three recordings and children over 2 years should be recorded annually. Measurements should be plotted on (New 9) centile charts as part of a screen for growth failure. All children below the second centile should be reviewed by the GP, especially if the child has tall parents. The GP should also review all children crossing a centile, even if still within normal limits or if there is parental concern. All children below the 0.4th centile should be referred for a specialist opinion. Normal growth velocity of children over 2 years is 5 cm/year and is calculated by the formula: (increase in height in cm × 12)/number of months = cm/year.

3.5 ABE

If a child has an unkempt, frightened withdrawn appearance with 'frozen watchfulness' and possibly, failure to thrive, developmental delay and evidence of physical injury then practitioners should have a high degree of suspicion of abuse. An acute hyphaema (ie blood in the anterior chamber of the eye) may result from serious shaking and scalds over both buttocks are typical of a forced immersion. However, a midclavicular fracture in a 10-day-old infant may have resulted from a difficult delivery and although a green/yellow bruise is evidence of an old injury (more precise estimation from the colour of the bruise is notoriously unreliable), this is a common finding in an active toddler.

3.6 AB

Tinea pedis (athlete's foot) is common in adolescents, leading to itchy, macerated and peeling skin between the toes with an unpleasant odour. Tinea capitis (scalp ringworm) is often caused by *Trichophyton* and results in hair loss, circular patches of alopecia with scaling skin and broken hairs. Tinea corporis results in itching with or without scaly circular lesions anywhere on the skin. There may also be small vesicles at the periphery. The differential diagnosis includes eczema, psoriasis and the 'Herald patch' of pityriasis rosea. *Microsporum canis* infections fluoresce under Wood's light. Fungal infections are identified by examining skin scrapings and plucked hairs under the microscope for hyphae and spores.

Small areas may be treated with topical clotrimazole cream; however, large areas require a 4- to 6-week course of oral griseofulvin. The rest of the family (including pets) should be examined and treated as necessary.

3.7 BC

One per cent of hips are found to be unstable at birth and are more common on the left (60%). Risk factors include female sex (80%), family history, breech delivery, first child and history of oligohydramnios. Screening involves the Ortolani–Barlow manoeuvre with USS of suspicious joints (X-rays are unhelpful before 6 weeks). If these tests are positive, neonates should be splinted in abduction for 6–12 weeks with clinical and radiological follow-up at 3, 6 and 12 months. Most hips will stabilise with conservative methods; however, those with persistent instability will need surgery. This is more likely if initial treatment was delayed.

3.8 ABC

Normal arterial $PaCO_2$ is an ominous sign, as a patient with acute asthma usually hyperventilates and consequently has low arterial $PaCO_2$. A normal $PaCO_2$ implies the patient is becoming exhausted and beginning to hypoventilate and may indicate impending respiratory arrest as the $PaCO_2$ continues to climb. The BTS guidelines define severe acute asthma as being: too breathless to talk; too breathless to feed; respirations > 50 breaths/minute, pulse > 140 beats/minute and a peak expiratory flow rate (PEFR) $< 50\%$ predicted or best. Other features of life-threatening asthma include PEFR $< 33\%$ predicted or best, a silent chest or poor respiratory effort, agitation, fatigue, decreased level of consciousness and central cyanosis. (NB Peripheral cyanosis is of little predictive value as it may be affected by numerous causes including the weather!) Pulsus paradoxus of > 20 mmHg is said to indicate severe acute asthma, although this is a difficult sign to demonstrate and is rarely used. Pectus carinatum, however, is a sign of chronic asthma and has no significance regarding the severity of an acute attack.

3.9 BC

Acute epiglottitis is caused by *Haemophilus influenzae* type b. It generally occurs between 2 and 6 years of age and the diagnosis is made from the history and classic clinical appearance. Within a few hours of developing a sore throat the child becomes hot, toxic, drools due to difficulty swallowing, and is unable to speak and is anxious. The child is dyspnoeic, has inspiratory stridor, subcostal recession and typically holds their head in hyperextension to maximise the airway. There is usually no cough. Anything that may increase the child's distress should be avoided as this may precipitate a respiratory arrest requiring an emergency attempt at endotracheal intubation by junior staff. This includes unnecessary investigations, such as a lateral neck X-ray, and examination of the throat is absolutely contraindicated. If the condition is suspected an experienced anaesthetist should called to perform an elective endotracheal intubation in a controlled environment, such as a theatre.

3.10 ABCDE

Common side-effects of phenytoin include nausea, vomiting, mental confusion, dizziness, headache and tremor. Coarse facies, acne, hirsutism and gingival hyperplasia are particularly undesirable in adolescent patients. Rarer side-effects include dyskinesias, SLE, erythema multiforme (Stevens–Johnson syndrome) and blood disorders. Plasma calcium may be lowered (rickets and osteomalacia). Ataxia, slurred speech, nystagmus and blurred vision are signs of overdosage.

3.11 BCE

Tics are defined as stereotypic, repetitive, involuntary movements. Simple developmental tics affect 15% of primary school children. They involve movements of the head, neck and shoulders (eg blinking, sniffing, shrugging) and are not generally of pathological significance. Most are usually outgrown by 4 years of age and rarely persist beyond adolescence. Tics may be familial in origin.

3.12 CD

The most common reason for a child to be admitted to hospital in the UK is for an acute exacerbation of asthma. Initial investigations should include PEFR in children older than 5 years; however, it is difficult to measure accurately in younger children and is therefore not a reliable measure of severity in this group. A chest X-ray is not required routinely and is only indicated if the diagnosis is in doubt or an associated severe infection or pneumothorax is clinically suspected. IV steroids should only be given with an acute exacerbation if the child is vomiting, otherwise oral preparations are sufficient. IV fluids should be restricted to two-thirds of normal maintenance, as increased secretion of antidiuretic hormone occurs with severe asthma resulting in fluid retention.

3.13 ABDE

The MMR vaccine is contraindicated in patients who are allergic to neomycin or kanamycin. In children who have had a previous anaphylactic reaction to egg, routine immunisation is not advised and should be discussed with a local paediatrician or immunisation co-ordinator. The MMR vaccine should not be given within 3 weeks of another live vaccine, as this results in a suboptimal response. Likewise, it is contraindicated in patients who have received an injection of immunoglobulin within 3 months, as no response will be mounted in the presence of immunoglobulin that may contain measles, mumps or rubella antibodies. Pregnancy should be avoided for at least 1 month after immunisation, which may well result in a rash with or without fever from about day 5–10 lasting approximately 2 days. It is therefore sensible to provide advice on temperature control at the time of vaccination.

3.14 BDE

An adverse obstetric history is a risk factor including previous ectopic pregnancy, abortion, antepartum haemorrhage, preterm labour, caesarean section, perinatal death or congenital abnormality. A birth interval of 18–36 months is associated with the lowest perinatal mortality rate, whereas an interval less than 12 months has the highest. Multiple pregnancy and maternal age greater than 35 years are also risk factors.

3.15 ACE

Plagiocephaly is associated with craniosynostosis and also with babies who have suffered damage to their sternomastoid muscle and consequently develop a sternomastoid tumour (which may present with torticollis). This pulls the head persistently to the affected side resulting in retarded facial growth on that side and hence facial asymmetry. A recent increase in the incidence may be attributable to the 'Back to Sleep' campaign to combat sudden infant death syndrome (SIDS). Advice on alternating the head position in the cot generally results in spontaneous improvement over time. If it is secondary to sternomastoid tumour it may also resolve, but may need physiotherapy if it persists. Later treatment involves division of the muscle at the distal end.

3.16 ACE

Common side-effects of carbamazepine include nausea and vomiting, dizziness, drowsiness, headache, ataxia (phenytoin and clonazepam also have these effects), confusion and agitation (in the elderly), visual disturbances, anorexia, diarrhoea or constipation. A mild transient erythematous rash may occur in a large number of patients (this may need discontinuation of the drug if it worsens). Leukopenia and other blood disorders (thrombocytopenia, agranulocytosis and aplastic anaemia) are also recognised. Rickets is a known side-effect of phenytoin and phenobarbitone while transient hair loss is typical of sodium valproate.

3.17 AC

Common side-effects of clonazepam are somnolence (and paradoxical hyperactivity), muscle hypotonia, fatigue, dizziness, co-ordination disturbances and hypersalivation in infancy. Rarer side-effects include blood disorders and abnormal liver function. Acne occurs with phenytoin and nystagmus with overdose. Reversible leukopenia is more typical of carbamazepine.

3.18 ACDE

Cystic fibrosis is an autosomal recessive disorder and affects approximately 1 in 2000 live births in the UK. Presenting features include meconium ileus, recurrent respiratory infection, failure to thrive, loose stools, steatorrhoea and malabsorption. Other associated features include rectal prolapse, short stature, delayed puberty, diabetes mellitus, chronic sinusitis and nasal polyps.

3.19 ABDE

3.20 ABD

Primary prevention is aimed at preventing the 'accident' from happening and includes speed limits, stair gates, teaching road safety and child-proof catches on cupboards. Secondary prevention aims to prevent injury should the 'accident' happen. Examples of secondary prevention include cycling helmets, seat belts, smoke alarms and fire extinguishers kept in the house. NB Child-resistant lids are a form of primary prevention as they prevent the child from reaching the drug; however, blister packs for prescription drugs merely limit the number of a tablets a child can get at in a given time and are therefore a form of secondary prevention. Tertiary prevention aims to limit the impact of an injury once the 'accident' has happened and includes teaching parents first aid skills and providing good access to the emergency services.

3.21 ABCD

Features of congenital rubella syndrome include deafness, eye defects (microphthalmia, cataract, retinopathy and glaucoma), cardiac defects (PDA, ASD and pulmonary stenosis), cerebral palsy, microcephaly, mental retardation and osteitis. Saddle nose is a feature of congenital syphilis.

3.22 AD

CHD has an incidence of 8 per 1000 live births with VSD being the most common. Acyanotic lesions (eg VSD, ASD, PDA and pulmonary stenosis) are approximately three times more common than cyanotic lesions (eg TGA and Fallot's) and generally have a better prognosis. Down's syndrome is associated with an increased incidence of VSD and ASD. Other risk factors for CHD include maternal drug and alcohol abuse, maternal diabetes, maternal infection (eg rubella), a positive family history and Turner's syndrome (eg coarctation). Indometacin is a prostaglandin synthetase inhibitor and may lead to premature closure of the ductus. In TGA, iv prostaglandin E is given to keep the ductus open until urgent catheterisation can be carried out. Definitive surgery is postponed until about 9–12 months.

3.23 CDE

Short-term fostering is usually less than 6 months, if a longer placement is required then adoption should be considered. Long-term fostering is preferred for older children, whereas adoption is more appropriate for younger children. Fostering is more likely to be successful if there are children of a similar age in the placement family. There is usually a limit of three foster children per family, however more may be fostered if they are all siblings. All children in long-term foster care require a 6-monthly medical examination and the GP has a vital role in co-ordinating services and ensuring continuing medical care.

3.24 B

Aerosol inhalers are appropriate for children over 10 years of age; however, if their technique is poor, then a spacer device, which allows inhaled drugs to be given adequately at any age, may be appropriate. A plastic coffee cup makes an adequate (and cheap) homemade 'back-up' spacer device by simply making a small hole in the base for the inhaler and then placing the rim firmly over the child's mouth and nose while the metered dose is given. Dry powder inhalers are suitable for a child over 5 years and oral salbutamol syrup is often prescribed in primary care for the treatment of infants and toddlers, although an inhaler plus spacer device may be more beneficial.

3.25 BCD

SIDS is defined as death of an infant or young child which is unexpected by history and in whom a thorough post-mortem fails to reveal an adequate explanation. The incidence varies worldwide with marked seasonal variation (increases in winter months) and is the leading cause of death in infants over 1 week of age. Risk factors include male sex, multiple births, low birth weight babies, associated respiratory infection, bottle feeding, social classes IV and V and the prone sleeping position (the supine position helps reduce the risk). A history of a sibling dying of SIDS increases the risk 10-fold, whereas maternal substance abuse increases the risk 30-fold. Management involves support and reassuring the parents they are not to blame. The need for a post-mortem should be explained and, if a twin, the sibling should be investigated and observed. The GP should visit the same day and follow up regularly over the next few weeks as once the acute shock is over, depression may ensue.

3.26 ABC

Of children with cystic fibrosis 95% have pancreatic insufficiency that results in steatorrhoea and fat-soluble vitamin (A, D, E and K) deficiency requiring supplementation. Consequently, children often have excellent appetites following treatment and undiagnosed, non-compliant or unwell children are often anorexic. The investigation of choice is the sweat test – to confirm the diagnosis three tests should be abnormal (ie sweat sodium > 70 mmol/l). Cystic fibrosis is a Caucasian disorder, it has a lower incidence in Afro-Caribbeans and is very rare in the Chinese. Cystic fibrosis causes male infertility but not impotence.

3.27 CDE

Routine screening of all children for VUR does not fulfil Wilson and Jungner's criteria for cost-effectiveness. However, it is vital to investigate all children presenting with a UTI as approximately 35% will have VUR and about 35% of these go on to develop renal scarring, although the risks reduce with age and degree of reflux. Reflux nephropathy is the most important cause of renal hypertension and chronic renal failure in childhood. A micturating cysto-urethrogram is the investigation of choice for diagnosis, with renal growth and morphology being monitored by serial USS.

VUR is graded as follows:

Grade I: reflux into lower end of ureter without dilatation

Grade II: urine refluxes into the kidney on micturition only

Grade III: reflux enters kidney during both bladder filling and voiding

Grade IV: reflux with dilatation of the ureter or renal pelvis.

Management of grade IV VUR is debatable and should be referred for a urological opinion. Conservative medical management may be all that is required, however surgical re-implantation of the ureters is an option.

3.28 BCD

In spastic diplegia the legs are more severely affected than the arms; in spastic hemiplegia there is asymmetrical tone and reduced movements on the affected side (arm relatively weaker than leg) with the limbs on the affected side being smaller, colder and spastic – although almost all children are usually walking by school age. Spastic hemiplegia may result from an infarct of the cortex or internal capsule and only about 30% have an IQ less than 70.

3.29 ACDE

There may be general signs of sexual abuse (eg superficial injuries, recurrent UTI); perineal signs (eg soreness, vaginal discharge); and behavioural signs (eg sexualised behaviour, depression, bedwetting, drug dependence). Chlamydia and genital warts are the common sexually transmitted diseases (STDs) in child sex abuse. HIV infection in children is generally through vertical transmission; however, it may occur through sexual abuse. Anal fissures, skin tags, reflex dilatation and perianal bruising also rouse suspicion of, but are not pathognomonic of, sexual abuse.

3.30 BCE

ARF is a sudden disturbance of renal function resulting in decreased urine output with rising serum urea and creatinine. There are three main causes of ARF:

- prerenal: due to hypovolaemia (eg burns) or hypotension (eg septicaemia)
- renal: eg haemolytic uraemic syndrome, acute glomerulonephritis and nephrotoxins (ie gentamicin)
- post-renal: due to congenital (eg urethral valves) or acquired (eg renal calculi) obstructive uropathy.

Management involves resuscitation, fluid restriction, correction of electrolytes, iv antibiotics if septic, a high-calorie/low-protein diet (total parenteral nutrition (TPN) may be necessary) and possibly dialysis. Indications for dialysis include a diuretic-resistant hypervolaemia with hypertension and pulmonary oedema, a plasma urea > 54 mmol/l, hyperkalaemia, metabolic acidosis or a dialysable nephrotoxin. ARF may be complicated by convulsions and tetany, which are secondary to the associated hypocalcaemia and hypomagnesaemia.

3.31 BDE

The BTS guidelines define severe acute asthma as: too breathless to talk; too breathless to feed; respiration > 50 breaths/minute; pulse > 140 beats/minute; and a PEFR < 50% predicted or best. Life-threatening features are defined as: PEFR < 33% predicted or best; cyanosis, a silent chest, or poor respiratory effort; fatigue or exhaustion; and agitation or decreased level of consciousness. Children with severe attacks may not appear distressed and assessment in the young may be difficult. Therefore, the presence of any of the above features should alert the doctor.

3.32 ADE

Infantile colic characteristically presents with paroxysmal crying and 'pulling up' of the legs and infrequently lasts beyond 3 months of age. There is no known cause and a child should only be labelled as having colic by exclusion of all other likely and serious diagnoses. Although there is no clinically effective treatment, the child may require a social admission to hospital to break the cycle of stressed mother and crying baby.

3.33 ABCE

UTIs are more common in boys in the first month of life and become more common in girls from about 6 months. *E. coli* is responsible for approximately 80% of cases. Other causative organisms include *Klebsiella*, *Streptomyces albus* and *Proteus*. In neonates most UTIs are haematogenous in origin, whereas in older infants and children infection generally ascends from the native bowel flora. About 35% of all children presenting with a UTI have VUR, with 45% having some structural or functional abnormality of their urinary tract (90% if < 2 years and 60% if < 5 years). Significant bacteriuria from a normal mid-stream urine (MSU) or clean catch has > 105 CFU of bacteria/ml; however, a suprapubic aspirate requires > 103 CFU of bacteria/ml only.

3.34 ABCDE

Primary generalised tonic-clonic epilepsy is rare, has no known cause and typically presents after 5 years of age. There is usually no aura, although these do occur in partial seizures with secondary generalisation. Features include an initial tonic spasm associated with collapse, loss of consciousness and cyanosis lasting more than 60 seconds. This is usually followed by clonic spasms with incontinence and tongue biting lasting more than 3 minutes. The ensuing postictal phase or coma gradually resolves over several minutes to hours with headache, drowsiness, confusion, myalgia and automatism. Complications include status epilepticus which is a fit (or consecutive fits without complete recovery between) lasting more than 30 minutes. The EEG may be normal between seizures or show bursts of spike waves. During the tonic phase, diffuse runs of spike waves occur with slow waves alternating with spike waves in the clonic phase. First-line treatment is carbamazepine, with 70% of patients being fit-free on monotherapy alone. Second-line agents include lamotrigine or valproate with phenytoin and phenobarbitone being third-line agents. After 15 years, 80% will remain in remission off treatment altogether.

3.35 BCDE

NAI should be suspected when there is a delay in presentation of the child with an inadequate or inconsistent explanation of the symptoms or lesions. An unusual parental attitude, such as over-protection or alternatively appearing unconcerned, should also cause concern. Accidental skull fractures tend to be single, linear, narrow and parietal with rarely any associated intracranial injury. A depressed skull fracture is therefore highly suspicious, as is a fractured tibia in a non-ambulant child of 6 months. Black eyes are difficult to get except by a punching injury, consequently unilateral, but particularly bilateral, black eyes are suggestive of abuse.

3.36 A

Before adoption proceeds informed consent from both natural parents (or mother if the child is illegitimate) is desirable. However, it is not needed if they cannot be found, are incapable of agreeing, have abandoned or neglected the child, have persistently ill-treated the child and are unlikely ever to be able to look after the child adequately. Applicants wanting to adopt a child must be aged 21 or more and adoption is arranged through registered agencies. The child must live with the adoptive parents for 3 months before the order is finalised, at which time all rights and responsibilities pass irreversibly to the adoptive parents. The original parents have no right of access. The adopted child takes on the nationality of their adoptive parents and has no claim to maintenance or inheritance from their original parent(s). At age 18 years an adopted child is entitled to their original birth certificate.

3.37 ABCE

Rickets is the inadequate mineralisation of new bone in developing bones (osteomalacia in adults). It is most commonly secondary to vitamin D deficiency (eg diet, malabsorption or lack of exposure to sunlight). Other associations include chronic renal failure and anticonvulsant therapy, as phenytoin and phenobarbitone induce liver enzymes resulting in accelerated breakdown of cholecalciferol to its inactive metabolite. Inherited causes include vitamin D-dependent (autosomal recessive) and vitamin D-resistant (X-linked dominant trait) rickets.

Clinical features include frontal bossing, kyphoscoliosis, hypotonia, swelling at the wrist and costochondral junctions ('rickety rosary'). Bow legs (genu varum) are more usual in toddlers, whereas knock-knees (genu valgum) are typical of older children. Tetany and convulsions secondary to hypocalcaemia may occur rarely.

Treatment of nutritional rickets involves parental education and high-dose vitamin D supplements for 4–6 weeks, followed by a low dose until biochemical and radiological resolution.

3.38 ACDE

3.39 ABDE

Acute lymphoblastic leukaemia has a 50–75% 5-year disease-free survival rate, but approximately 10% relapse within the first year. Poor prognostic features include age $<$ 2 years or $>$ 10 years, a presenting WCC $>$ 20,000/mm^3, T- or B-cell surface markers, elevated acid phosphatase in T-cell leukaemia, an anterior mediastinal mass or CNS signs at presentation. Being Caucasian is a good prognostic factor.

3.40 AD

Crohn's disease is characterised by inflammation of the whole thickness of the bowel, especially the terminal ileum and proximal colon, the rectum is usually spared. The incidence has increased over the past 20–30 years and now affects about 5 per 100, 000 individuals. Presenting features include failure to thrive, mouth ulcers, anorexia, abdominal pain and diarrhoea. Other non-gastrointestinal features include erythema nodosum, arthritis, digital clubbing and anaemia. Investigations include a malabsorption and infection screen, endoscopy, biopsy and barium meal, which may reveal the characteristic 'string sign', 'skip lesion' and 'rose thorn ulcers' seen in Crohn's disease.

Ulcerative colitis classically has diffuse inflammation and ulceration of the entire rectal and colonic mucosa and is also associated with an incidence of 5 per 100, 000. It typically presents within the first 12 months or around 10 years of age with intermittent episodes of abdominal pain and bloody diarrhoea. Other features include lethargy, fever, clubbing, mouth ulcers, anaemia, arthritis, short stature, erythema nodosum and toxic dilatation of the colon. Investigations include malabsorption and infection screens, double contrast barium enema, colonoscopy and biopsies.

Management of both conditions involves a high-energy, low-fibre diet with vitamin supplements and drugs (eg mesalazine or sulfasalazine) associated with immunosuppressive agents, such as steroids. Surgery is indicated in Crohn's only if there are complications such as bowel obstruction or perforation. However, in ulcerative colitis, surgery may be required for failure to respond to conservative treatment, toxic dilatation, severe gastro-intestinal bleeding, perforation and ultimately as prophylaxis against its associated increased risk of malignancy.

3.41 BD

Precocious puberty is defined as the onset of sexual maturation before 8 years in a girl and 9 years in a boy. It is at least four times more common in girls and usually no cause is found. However, in boys it is essential to investigate as in 80–90% of cases a cause is found (eg intracranial tumour). The most important sequela is decreased final height, as the initial associated growth spurt is short lived and the advanced bone age results in early epiphyseal fusion.

Important investigations include skull X-ray, bone age, CT scan of the head, urinary 17-ketosteroids, pelvic USS and thyroid function tests (TFTs). Management involves referral to a specialist for treatment aiming to achieve continually high levels of synthetic gonadotrophin-releasing hormone (GnRH) analogues in the circulation. This 'non-pulsatile' regimen paradoxically suppresses the secretion of pituitary gonadotrophins, which reverses gonadal and slows skeletal maturation. Treatment should be continued until the average age of puberty (ie 11 years) and parents should be reassured that the child will develop normally.

Features of McCune–Albright syndrome include polyosteotic fibrous dysplasia of bone, irregular areas of skin pigmentation, facial asymmetry with or without precocious puberty. Coeliac disease is associated with delayed puberty.

3.42 B

Bow legs are normal in infants and usually correct by 3 years of age. Knock knees (genu valgum) are normal up to approximately 5 years. Predisposing conditions include osteogenesis imperfecta, rickets, Blount's disease (infantile tibia vara) and chondrodysplasia. Genu varum also results from medial tibial torsion; this usually spontaneously corrects within 5 years and no treatment is required. However, forward bowing is pathological (eg rickets) and active management is essential. Osgood–Schlatter's disease occurs with inflammation of the tibial tuberosity at the insertion of the patella tendon and results in painful knees. Neither bow legs nor knock knees is a feature, although the latter is a common sequela of poliomyelitis.

3.43 BDE

A normal 18-month-old infant can kick a ball forward; this develops between 15 months and 2 years. They can walk backwards from about 1 year and can climb upstairs holding on, but use two feet per step. They cannot balance on one foot as this develops later at around 22 months to 3 years. 'Bottom-shufflers' may be delayed walkers although most infants walk well by 14 months.

3.44 B

Neither HIV nor AIDS is a notifiable disease. The risk of vertical transmission in Europe is between 13% and 25% and has been shown to decrease with antiviral drugs in pregnancy and caesarean section, although this figure is much higher in Africa. Testing neonates for the presence of HIV antibodies is not helpful in excluding a congenital infection because of the transmission of maternal antibodies. However, P24 antigen and polymerase chain reaction are of use. Although the risk of transmission via breast milk is small, where safe alternatives are available breast-feeding should be avoided. However, in developing countries the risks of breast-feeding far outweigh the benefits of the alternatives and should therefore be encouraged. NB HIV is a positive indication for pneumococcal vaccination.

3.45 BE

A normal 3-year-old is usually 'dry' both day and night. They can feed, wash and dress themselves without supervision, including donning shoes, but are unable to manage complex buckles or laces. They will interact with other children in both imaginary and non-imaginary play.

Extending Matching Answers

3.46 Respiratory distress in the newborn

1 I – Surfactant deficient lung disease (hyaline membrane disease)

While all of the options are possible I is the most likely from the information given. Pulmonary hypoplasia and persistent pulmonary hypertension of the newborn are also possible but the most common cause of RDS at birth at 24/40 is hyaline membrane disease (HMD).

2 H – Pulmonary hypoplasia

Since the fetal lungs require amniotic fluid to develop properly, rupture of membranes at 16 weeks will lead to oligohydramnios and subsequent pulmonary hypoplasia. Erythromycin reduces incidence of congenital pneumonia. HMD is less likely at 33/40.

3 J – Transient tachypnoea of newborn

Transient tachypnoea of newborn is the most likely diagnosis as caesarean sections don't provide stimulation for absorption of lung fluid. This is the most likely diagnosis if there was an uncomplicated antenatal course.

3.47 Genetic diseases

1 A – Autosomal dominant

Achondroplasia is an autosomal dominant condition, however 90% of cases occur as a result of a new mutation.

2 C – Autosomal recessive

Sickle cell disease is a good example of an autosomal recessive inherited condition. The chance of inheritance of the disease (HbSS) is 1 in 4 if both parents are heterozygotes (HbSs). The expression of the gene in the population is increasing as the heterozygote form (sickle cell trait) provides resistance to malaria in endemic countries.

3 J – X-linked recessive

Duchenne muscular dystrophy occurs in 1 in 3000 of live male births. There is a significant new mutation rate (30%). The underlying abnormality is a decreased production of dystrophin. Presentation is usually in early childhood. There may be a history of delay in walking and a tendency to fall. Difficulty in getting up from a sitting position can be demonstrated (Gower's sign). Hip flexion contractures and calf hypertrophy lead to toe walking. Of those affected 90% are wheel-chair bound by puberty and 30% have some mental disability.

3.48 Blood disorders

1 E – G-6-PD deficiency

G-6-PD deficiency is more common in people of Mediterranean origin (up to 35%). Haemolysis can be triggered by a number of factors (favism, antimalarials, sulphonamides, etc) – in this case probably nitrofurantoin given frequently for UTIs. The picture is of a haemolytic anaemia – there is a very good reticulocyte response showing that bone marrow production is good. Thalassaemia is unlikely as this is presented as an acute problem.

2 H – Immune-mediated thrombocytopenia purpura

This is a typical picture of immune-mediated thrombocytopenia purpura. The low platelet count is due to peripheral destruction of platelets not failure of production (megakaryocytes are precursors of platelets in the bone marrow).

3 G – Henoch–Schönlein purpura

The distribution of the rash is consistent with Henoch–Schönlein purpura. In a well child, with normal platelets and clotting, meningococcal septicaemia is less likely; however, it should always be considered.

3.49 Infant nutrition

1 E -- 1 year

Pasta contains gluten, which should be avoided until 1 year of age.

2 B – 4 months

Baby rice is a good food to start weaning. Weaning should start at 4–6 months (although the WHO recommends exclusive breast-feeding until 6 months old).

3 C – 7 months

3.50 Systemic diseases

1 C – Kawasaki's disease

The major criteria of Kawasaki's disease are: cervical lymph-adenopathy (>2 cm), non-purulent conjunctivitis, mucositis, high spiking fever for > 5 days, polymorphous rash/extremity change.

2 B – Dermatomyositis

The age of the girl makes some diagnoses more likely than others (eg dermatomyositis, SLE). However, the rash affecting the eyelids is characteristic of dermatomyositis, along with the raised CK. The pain in the knees and legs is due to the myositis and not an arthritis per se.

3 E – Pauci-articular juvenile idiopathic arthritis

dsDNA –ve makes SLE unlikely, ASOT –ve renders rheumatic fever unlikely. The clinical picture fits with that of juvenile idiopathic arthritis (previously juvenile chronic arthritis). This is pauci-articular as it involves four or less joints. The ANA +ve means that there is a high risk of iridocyclitis and the patient must be screened for this.

3.51 Genetic syndromes

1 G – Pierre Robin syndrome

These are typical features for Pierre Robin syndrome. The mandibular hypoplasia causes a degree of glossoptosis (tongue obstructing airway posteriorly). These infants should be nursed prone and may often require a naso-pharyngeal airway to be used until the face/jaw has grown sufficiently. If there is an associated microcephaly then the child may have some mental disability, otherwise intelligence is normal.

2 E – Noonan's syndrome

Noonan's syndrome has a similar phenotype to Turner's syndrome, but can occur in both sexes. There is often a degree of learning difficulties. Noonan's syndrome has an association with right-sided cardiac defects (especially pulmonary stenosis).

3 D – Fragile X syndrome

In any child with marked behavioural or learning difficulties, if no other cause is obvious, fragile X should always be considered. Fragile X is the second most common genetic cause (trinucleotide repeat sequences on the X chromosome) for learning difficulties in males (Down's syndrome being the most common). Phenotypically, children with fragile X have large ears, long noses and high foreheads. Testicular volume is markedly increased.

3.52 Vaccinations

1 H – Salk polio vaccine

OPV is excreted in the stools for approximately 4 weeks after inoculation. This means there is a risk of immunocompromised children (eg premature neonates) being infected with polio vaccine. On SCBU neonates should be given inactivated polio (Salk type). If the baby is close to going home the oral live vaccine (Sabin type) can be given as they leave.

2 A – Acellular pertussis vaccine

Prolonged (> 4 hours) inconsolable crying is classed as a generalised adverse reaction to immunisation. Prolonged crying is mostly attributable to whole cell pertussis vaccine, and so immunisation with acellular pertussis vaccine is advisable subsequently. If there is the same reaction to acellular pertussis then omission of the pertussis vaccine is recommended the next time. All indications and contraindications for immunisation are to be found in *Immunisation against Infectious Disease 1996 – 'The Green Book'*, this is also available on the Department of Health website (www.doh.gov.uk initially accessed 1 October 2003).

3 B – Conjugate pneumococcal vaccine

Any child or adult who has had a splenectomy (or splenic compromise as in sickle disease) is at risk of infection from encapsulated organisms. The younger the child the more at risk they are. In a 1-year-old the conjugate vaccine should be given; this provides protection against seven pneumococcal serotypes. As the vaccine is conjugated it provokes a better immune response than the unconjugated variety. It must not be forgotten that once the child is over 2 years the unconjugated vaccine should be given as it provides a wider cover (30–40 pneumococcal serotypes).

3.53 Psychiatric disorders

1 D – Autism

Autism is an increasing problem. It was first described by Kanner in 1943. It is a triad of communication difficulties, socialisation problems and attention problems. This 3-year-old shows poor language skills and poor eye contact (socialisation problem). The features of autism are mostly present before 2 years of age but the diagnosis may not necessarily be made at that time. The language difficulties can be profound and up to 30% of autistic children may never develop language. Treatment modalities include speech and language therapy, behavioural therapy to improve socialisation and attention.

2 G – Psycho-social deprivation

In a child who was previously thriving but is now growth faltering, and who has some developmental delay, the diagnosis of psycho-social deprivation must always be considered. This is a diagnosis of exclusion, once organic causes have been ruled out. In this case there are other warning sign of this diagnosis – she has missed some immunisations, she will play games (so probably has no socialisation difficulties) and her dentition is poor, a possible sign of neglect.

3 H – Post-traumatic stress disorder

Post-traumatic stress disorder, although still uncommon, is an increasing diagnosis in paediatric psychiatry. The trauma of the sexual assault has led to the behavioural problems in this girl. Post-traumatic stress disorder can be due to sexual assault, physical assault or indeed any experience of very traumatic situations (eg refugees from a conflict zone). It can present in a myriad of ways: concentration difficulties, mood instability, aggression, flashbacks, sleep disturbance, anxiety, depression and parasuicide. Cognitive–behavioural therapy and counselling may help the disclosure of the trigger, and provide effective results.

3.54 Special investigations

1 D – Echocardiogram

The single most important late complication of Kawasaki disease is development of coronary artery aneurysms. An echocardiogram, in skilled hands, is an easy, simple and effective way of detecting aneurysms. An angiogram is sometimes performed in tertiary paediatric cardiac centres, to further demonstrate aneurysms seen on the echocardiogram.

2 C – CT

Any seizure following a head injury is an indication for further imaging. A skull X-ray may reveal a skull fracture, but given the fact that there has been a seizure brain imaging is required. CT scans of the brain are quick to do and readily available and are the investigation of choice in the NICE guidelines for the management of a head injury.

3 B – Bone scan

The concern in this child is that there may be an underlying osteomyelitis. A plain film may reveal some periosteal reaction, but only if the infection has been present for over 1 week. A bone scan is the investigation of choice. An osteomyelitis will show as a 'hot spot' at the point where the infection is. MRI is now being increasingly used to look for periosteal and intramedullary oedema.

Best of Five Answers

3.55 B: Intussusception

'The most important to exclude' – Intussusception is the only one that is potentially life-threatening. The others are, of course, possible diagnoses but not immediately life-threatening.

3.56 C: Parainfluenza virus type 3

These symptoms are classic of croup. The most common cause is parainfluenza 3.

3.57 C: Over-feeding

While all of the answers would cause the listed symptoms, pyloric stenosis, jejunal stenosis and gastro-enteritis would be very unlikely in a thriving child. The daily volume of feed is quite substantial (1200 ml) and in a 5-kg baby would work out to 240 ml/kg per day!

3.58 D: Increase in testicular volume

Increase in testicular volume is the first sign of puberty in boys (from 10 years). Voice change occurs at around 14 years. Peak height velocity is when testicular volume reaches 10 ml (pubic hair stage 4). There is a wide range in times of onset of the stages in individuals.

(A good reference for sequence of development is Marshall, W.A. and Tanner, J.M. 1970, Variations in the pattern of pubertal changes in boys. *Archives of Diseases in Childhood*, 45 (239),13–23.)

3.59 D: A 7-day course of oral erythromycin

In a child with no respiratory distress there is no need to admit unless oral antibiotics cannot be tolerated. BTS guidelines for community-acquired pneumonia in children suggest the use of a macrolide antibiotic as a first line in the over-fives if *Mycoplasma* is a possible causative organism. If, however, there are features that would suggest pneumococcal chest infection (focal consolidation/signs) then amoxicillin is the suggested first-line treatment.

3.60 A: Retro-pharyngeal abscess

Stridor indicates an upper airway problem. Croup is less likely in an unwell child, especially if there has been a preceding tonsillitis. Epiglottitis would be surprising in a child immunised against Hib, but it is recognised. Bacterial tracheitis is indeed a possibility but with a preceding tonsillitis a retro-pharyngeal abscess is more likely.

3.61 C: Prescribe her the OCP if she meets the Gillick criteria

Gillick competence is important to understand. Lord Fraser held that a girl under 16 years of age could be prescribed the OCP if the following criteria could be met:

1. The girl can understand, retain and make informed decisions on the information given to her.
2. That, despite discussion, she will definitely not involve her parents.
3. If she is going to have sexual intercourse whether the OCP is prescribed or not.
4. If the OCP is NOT prescribed it will be detrimental to her health.
5. If it is in her best interests.

There is now a move away from calling these criteria 'Gillick Competence' to 'Fraser Competent'.

3.62 B: Eyes rolling back followed by a 3-minute generalised tonic-clonic seizure. Drowsy afterwards for 1 hour

Typical features of a febrile convulsion are: age 6 months to 6 years and febrile (or rising temperature) at time of convulsion. Generalised tonic-clonic seizure lasting up to 10 minutes with a post-ictal phase afterwards. Eyes rolling back and incontinence are often seen. Answer A gives focal features with secondary generalisation – this is sometimes seen in febrile convulsions but is not typical. Answer C is again possible for a febrile convulsion but is more likely to be an absence. The duration of the seizures in D and E means that these are not typical.

3.63 C: Survival at this gestation is generally poor, and survivors may have long-term problems – (*then discuss with her the option of not resuscitating if the baby is in a poor condition*)

Discussion of potential morbidity and mortality with parents in threatened premature labour is difficult but very important. If there is a threatened delivery at 23 weeks of gestation it is important to discuss with the parents the possibility of not resuscitating if the condition of the baby is poor or the gestation looks to be earlier, as the outcome is likely to be very poor. It is useful to give parents morbidity and mortality figures – either national figures from the EPICURE study (*Pediatrics,* Oct. 2000, 106(4),659–71) or, preferably, the figures for your own unit.

3.64 A: Six-word vocabulary

Six-word vocabulary: by 2 years

Greater than 100-word vocabulary: 2≥ years

2–3 word phrases: by 25 months

Tuneful babbling: by 8 months

Sing nursery rhymes: by 3 years

3.65 E: It is probable that there will be no significant long-term effects but his development will be closely followed just in case

Grading of intraventricular haemorrhage:

Grade 1: Ependymal (germinal matrix)

Grade 2: Intraventricular without ventricular dilatation

Grade 3: Intraventricular with ventricular dilatation

Grade 4: Parenchymal

Prognosis depends on grade of bleed. Grades 1 and 2 have a good prognosis with no long-term effects. In Grade 3 there may be possible impairment on the contralateral side depending on degree of progression of dilatation and in Grade 4 likely motor impairment on contralateral side.

3.66 E: Reassure him and contact the school (with his consent) about the bullying

Gynaecomastia is not uncommon in puberty in boys and resolves spontaneously. Bullying is not acceptable and schools have very good anti-bullying policies. Surgical reduction is a last resort in gynaecomastia that doesn't resolve. Psychological support may be useful but will not stop the bullying per se.

3.67 C: Treat those contacts as advised by the CCDC

While it is within the remit of the CCDC – part of the public health department– to contact, trace and treat the necessary family members, it is good practice to liaise with them and treat the contacts at risk. This is easier for the acute clinicians to do as the contacts (usually family members) are often with the unwell child.

3.68 E: Tibial intra-osseous needle insertion

APLS recommendations indicate that tibial inter-osseus needle insertion is a quick and easy method of securing venous access in an arrested child. The other methods are satisfactory but in a collapsed child may be difficult and time consuming to insert.

3.69 C: Torted hydatid of Morgagni

The most likely diagnosis is a torted cyst of Morgagni (an embryonic remnant on the poles of the testes). However, the most important diagnosis to exclude is testicular torsion and so most will undergo surgical exploration. Mumps orchitis is rare now due to MMR. Infertility secondary to mumps orchitis is rare (<1%).

3.70 C: Advise applying 1% hydrocortisone cream bd for 1/52

The only medical indication for circumcision is balanitis xeroderma obliterans (BXO). A non-retractile foreskin is not uncommon until puberty. The adhesions may be released with some weak steroid cream. Ballooning of the foreskin is not a problem in itself.

3.71 B: Carbamazepine

Carbamazepine is a good first-line anticonvulsant. Plasma levels are easily monitored if control is not achieved. Carbamazepine is not as hepatotoxic as sodium valproate, and is less cardiotoxic than phenytoin (which also has zero-order kinetics making dose titration difficult). Diazepam prn is not a realistic treatment as the aim is to prevent seizures – not to treat them when they happen.

3.72 A: Use aqueous cream instead of soap, advise using a greasier emollient and try an antihistamine at night

Treatment of eczema can be problematic. It is worthwhile giving parents advice about simple, everyday measures that can improve the eczema: using non-biological washing powder; wearing cotton clothes as opposed to artificial fibres; and not using soaps or shampoos. Use of a bath oil (eg Oilatum) is beneficial and aqueous cream can be used as 'soap' to good effect. Regular emollient use is important, however, parents can find using very greasy products hard work as it involves a lot of washing of clothes. The aim is to keep the skin from feeling dry at any time of day. Sedating with older types of antihistamines at night do not help to reduce itching but used occasionally in large doses provide a sedative effect which may improve sleep. Once all these measures are in use but the eczema is still not controlled then escalation of treatment would be appropriate. There is no evidence for the benefit of topical antibiotics.

3.73 B: Micturating cystourethrogram

In an infant who has had a confirmed UTI and pevi-calyceal dilatation on USS, a micturating cystourethrogram is important to look for VUR. If present, VUR greatly increases the risk for renal scarring and so prophylactic antibiotics are extremely important to prevent this.

3.74 C: Referral to maxillofacial surgery for I&D

She has an abscess that has developed secondary to caries in her lower left 'E'. She has lymphadenitis secondary to this and since the swelling is fluctuant probably there is an abscess there. If there is a large (>1 cm) abscess present then the treatment is I&D with post-operative antibiotics. Antibiotics as a first line may reduce the infection but will not treat it completely if large. In the case of a small periodental/dental abscess then a course of oral antibiotics may treat the abscess, but advice to see a GDP should be reinforced.

NOTES FOR THE CLINICAL EXAMINATION FOR THE DCH

INTRODUCTION

It is important to read the College guidelines for the clinical part of the DCH examination. These can be obtained from the Royal College of Paediatrics and Child Health direct or downloaded from the College website. The guidelines set out the syllabus for the exam, the format, what is expected in the clinical section in general and specific guidelines relating to developmental assessment and child health surveillance.

It is of particular importance to read the following sections:

- Vision, visual disorders and visual testing in the DCH examination.
- Guidelines for hearing testing in the DCH clinicals.
- Language development guidelines.
- Child health surveillance: knowledge and standards for the DCH examination.
- Psychiatric guidelines.

The current format of the clinical exam (June 2004) is one Long Case, where 40 minutes is spent with the patient and 20 minutes with the examiners, followed by several Short Cases over 30 minutes, of which 10 minutes is devoted to developmental assessment, including the testing of vision and hearing. It is important to check with the college for changes particularly in view of recent changes to the written part of the exam.

The guidelines state that standard equipment appropriate for the examination will be provided. A stethoscope should be taken. You may prefer to take other objects with which you are familiar, such as an ophthalmoscope and developmental assessment kit.

Remember that the clinical examination tests your ability to:

- take a good case history
- perform a competent physical examination
- recognise abnormal physical signs
- assess growth and development
- assess the special senses
- assess psychiatric status.

THE LONG CASE

It is essential to get a clear medical history but also to concentrate on the social, behavioural, family and educational issues of the case. Use a checklist to make sure you don't miss out anything out:

- presenting complaint
- history of presenting complaint
- past medical history including birth history
- immunisations
- developmental history including behaviour and educational issues
- drugs history and allergies
- social history
- family history
- review of systems to check you haven't missed anything out.

Perform a complete physical examination including assessment of growth and development. Practise:

- seeing the child in the appropriate time
- presenting; and think out and practice answers to questions on the long case
- problem-orientated presentation.

This means presenting the patient clearly, listing active and inactive problems with the aim of giving the examiner an overview of the case in the first few sentences. Allocate your time carefully allowing time to collect your thoughts, think about the case and prepare the case for presentation to the examiners.

Examples of Problem-Orientated Presentation

Case 1

A 6-year-old girl presents with Down's syndrome. She has recently been diagnosed as hypothyroid. She is on treatment and well at the moment. Her other problems are:

- obesity
- constipation
- previous surgery for Hirschsprung's disease
- learning difficulties
- social and family issues.

It may be that the entire discussion focuses on the learning difficulties and how her schooling is sorted out. This includes:

- pre-school learning support including portage
- statement of special education needs
- review of special educational needs; requires knowledge of the assessment of children with special educational needs, which can be found in any of the standard community paediatric texts.

Alternatively, the examiner could focus on the medical complications seen in a child with Down's syndrome:

- cardiac problems
- hypothyroidism, other auto-immune problems
- hirschsprung's disease
- atlanto-axial instability
- leukaemia.

Alternatively, the examiner could spend most of the time discussing specific emotional issues:

- How have the child's problems affected the parents and the other siblings?
- What has been the effect on the integrity of the family unit?

Children with cerebral palsy are often seen and the case can be presented in a systematic and organised way in the same manner.

Case 2

An 8-year-old boy presents with cerebral palsy. He has spastic quadriplegia and is in a wheelchair. His main problems are:

- difficulties with feeding, poor weight gain and recurrent chest infections
- fits which are well controlled on anticonvulsant therapy
- joint contractures and poor mobility
- difficulties with schooling
- social and family issues.

It may be that you then go on to discuss either the medical aspects of this child's care or the multidisciplinary management. It is important to remember this list.

Professionals potentially involved in the multidisciplinary management of an 8-year-old with a spastic quadriplegia include:

- occupational therapist
- speech and language therapist
- dietician
- teacher
- educational psychologist
- social worker
- general practitioner
- community paediatrician
- orthopaedic surgeon.

This list could be applied to many other long cases.

Case 3

An 8-month-old infant presents with bronchopulmonary dysplasia. His condition is stable at the moment and his main problems are:

- chronic chest disease requiring home oxygen
- severe failure to thrive – nasogastric tube feed dependent
- pre-term – 25 weeks' gestation – with delayed motor development
- social problems.

The subsequent discussion may focus on one or all of these problems. Nutritional assessment will be of obvious concern and the reasons for his failure to thrive and the potential action that can be taken to overcome it may be discussed. Alternatively, the social situation could be focused on, with discussion about why there may be problems.

Examples of Long Cases

Any condition may be seen and it is important not to be too put off if you don't know that much about the case that you see. Concentrate on putting the case together and giving a well thought out multidisciplinary presentation.

Asthma

Cerebral palsy

Ex-premature baby with chronic lung disease

Cystic fibrosis

Spina bifida

Down's syndrome

Neurofibromatosis

Crohn's disease

Coeliac disease

Nephrotic syndrome

Chronic renal failure

Cyanotic congenital heart disease

Marfan's syndrome

Undiagnosed short stature

Prader–Willi syndrome

Muscular dystrophy.

THE SHORT CASES

It is essential to have a clear scheme for the examination of potential scenarios you might come across in the exam and a good knowledge base of the common conditions that you might see. This section outlines some of this with lists of commonly seen cases and should be used as a revision checklist in the preparation for the clinical part of the exam. The section does not duplicate the information listed in the DCH handbook relating to the examination of special senses (see above):

- Practise how you would deal with the listed common Short Cases.
- Practise interacting with the child and parent. Introduce yourself.
- Practise presentation skills. Make some initial comments. State what you can see; for example, if you think someone might have Down's syndrome say so. Otherwise the examiner won't know. The same goes for things like a nasogastric tube, drip etc. If you see something obvious say so.
- Practise talking through the examination.
- Team up with a like-minded candidate and practise presenting cases to each other.

Basic Format for the Clinical Examination

- be prepared to talk about your findings as you go on
- introduce yourself to the child and parent
- look
- feel
- listen
- describe your findings
- answer questions about them as you walk over to the next Short Case.

EXAMINATION OF CARDIOVASCULAR SYSTEM

Look

- Dysmorphic features, eg Down's syndrome (VSD), Turner's syndrome (coarctation), Noonan's syndrome (pulmonary stenosis)
- Is the child thriving?
- Respiratory distress, cyanosis.

Hands

- Pulse – brachial is better in babies, check for radio-femoral delay
- Clubbing
- Peripheral cyanosis.

Blood pressure

- Mention but don't necessarily do (but be prepared to if asked).

Face

- Anaemia
- Central cyanosis.

Neck

- Jugular venous pressure (JVP) (older child).

Scars

- Cardiac catheterisation scars
- Thoracotomy scars, eg shunt procedure, PDA ligation, coarctation repair
- Central sternotomy scars, eg corrective procedures (VSD repair, ASD repair, Tetralogy of Fallot repair, arterial switch for repair of TGA) or palliative procedures, eg shunt.

Palpation

- Apex beat – including localisation, presence of heaves – check for dextrocardia
- Thrills – include supra-sternal thrill and carotid thrill.

Auscultation

- Listen in the four areas
    - Mitral (apex)
    - Tricuspid (left sternal edge)
    - Aortic (right second intercostal space)
    - Pulmonary (left second intercostal space)
- Listen for radiation.

Heart sounds

- Are they present?
- Is the second heart sound normal – loud (pulmonary hypertension), split (ASD), single (aortic stenosis)?
- Click (aortic stenosis, pulmonary stenosis).

Murmurs

- Timing in relation to cardiac cycle
- Systolic/diastolic/continuous/mixed systolic and diastolic 'to and fro'
- Grade
- Site of maximal intensity, radiation (neck, axilla and back)
- Character
- Murmur enhancing moves – left lateral position, sitting forward.

Grading of murmurs

I	barely audible
II	medium intensity
III	loud but no thrill
IV	loud with a thrill
V	very loud but still requires stethoscope to be on the chest
VI	so loud, heard with stethoscope off the chest

Further examination

- Do not forget anything you may have left until the end, eg blood pressure, femoral pulses
- Listen to the back for murmurs
- Palpate the liver.

Common Short Cases – Cardiology

Innocent murmur

Ventricular septal defect

Atrioventricular septal defect

Atrial septal defect

Pulmonary stenosis

Aortic stenosis

Coarctation of the aorta

Dextrocardia – may be associated situs inversus

Cyanosed child who may or may not have had cardiac surgery

Eisenmenger's syndrome

Remember, children whose heart disease has been repaired may be seen and that chest wall scars may not be present; for example, a child who has had a balloon dilatation of pulmonary stenosis by cardiac catheter.

EXAMINATION OF RESPIRATORY SYSTEM

Look

- Is the child thriving, inhalers/nebulisers, pancreatic enzymes, peak flow meter, sputum pot?
- Is the child obviously hyperexpanded?
- Is the child in respiratory distress?

Hands

- Clubbing, cyanosis and anaemia
- Count pulse and respiratory rate.

Respiratory effort

- Examine for pectus excavatum and Harrison's sulcus
- Nasal flaring, recession, tracheal tug.

Mouth

- Central cyanosis.

Chest

- Scars
- Feel suprasternal notch for tracheal deviation, palpate apex beat (mediastinal shift)
- Percuss (anteriorly, posteriorly and laterally)
- Listen (anteriorly, posteriorly and laterally).

At the end of your examination

- Ask to examine the ears, nose and throat, see sputum specimen and perform peak flow measurement (if appropriate)
- Assess for tactile vocal fremitus, vocal resonance if appropriate (eg suspected consolidation)

In a baby it may be reasonable to change the order of examination to gain the maximum information.

Remember the common causes of clubbing

Congenital

Cyanotic congenital heart disease

Bacterial endocarditis

Cystic fibrosis

Bronchiectasis

Chronic active hepatitis

Inflammatory bowel disease.

Hyperexpansion

This implies chest disease and is an extremely important physical sign. Practise the assessment of hyperexpansion. Look from the front first and then assess by looking at the child from the side and examining antero-posterior diameter and its excursion during the respiratory phases. Comment on asymmetry if seen.

Causes of hyperexpansion – common conditions seen in the exam:

- Asthma
- Bronchopulmonary dysplasia – look for neonatal sequelae, eg head shape, chest drain/iv scars
- Cystic fibrosis
- Bronchiectasis.

Harrison's sulcus

Harrison's sulcus is visible as a bilateral fixed indrawing of the anterior portion of the lower ribs. It is caused by chronic airway obstruction encouraging excessive diaphragmatic use which causes deformity where the diaphragm inserts into the rib-cage. Its presence therefore suggests long-standing airway obstruction.

Pectus carinatum – prominent sternum

Pectus excavatum – sternal depression

Hyperexpanded chest plus clubbing implies cystic fibrosis or bronchiectasis

Hyperexpanded chest without clubbing implies asthma or bronchopulmonary dysplasia

GASTRO-INTESTINAL EXAMINATION

Remember gastro-intestinal examination will pick up gastro-intestinal, renal and haematological pathology.

Look

- Does the child look well?
- Normal or dysmorphic?
- Nasogastric tube, iv cannula?
- Well nourished (adequate exposure) – comment on nutritional status
- Mention the need to plot on a growth chart.

Hands

- Clubbing
- Koilonychia
- Palmar erythema
- Pallor.

Eyes

- Jaundice
- Anaemia.

Mouth

- Peri-oral pigmentation – Peutz–Jeghers syndrome
- Mouth ulceration
- Tongue – stomatitis
- Teeth.

Chest

- Spider naevi
- Gynaecomastia.

Abdomen

- Scars (laparoscope, groin, loin)
- Umbilical hernia
- Abnormal vessels – caput medusae (drain from the umbilicus)
- Distension
- Superficial palpation – all over once
- Deep palpation – all over once
- Liver
- Spleen
- Kidneys.

Further examination

This should be done as appropriate and depends on the previous findings. For example, it is not necessary to look for shifting dullness if the abdomen is not distended.

- Percussion
- Bowel sounds
- Abdominal distension – stand child up and look at buttocks as may also be wasted suggesting malabsorption
- Ascites – fluid thrill, shifting dullness – only if distended
- Can I see the back?
- Can I see the genitalia?
- Hernia orifices.

Common Short Cases – Gastro-intestinal Examination

Abdominal scars

Gastrostomy tube

Cystic fibrosis

Crohn's disease

Coeliac disease

Constipation

Umbilical hernia

Hepatomegaly, splenomegaly and hepatosplenomegaly

Glycogen and other storage disorders

Portal hypertension

Hereditary spherocytosis

Sickle cell disease

Thalassaemia

Mucopolysaccharidosis

Post Kasai for biliary atresia

Liver transplant

Nephrotic syndrome

Steroid toxicity

Renal masses.

EXAMINATION OF THE LIVER, SPLEEN AND KIDNEYS

- Important to do correctly
- Liver/spleen – start in right iliac fossa
- If organomegaly found, confirm with percussion – measure if appropriate.

Liver

- Edge – regular or irregular?
- Surface – smooth or nodular?
- Texture – firm or hard?
- Tenderness
- Is there a rub?
- Is there a bruit?

Spleen

- As above
- Hepatomegaly and ascites
- Associations, eg jaundice – hereditary spherocytosis.

Common Exam Questions

- How do you differentiate between a liver, spleen and kidney?
- Why is it a liver?
- Why is it a spleen?

Liver

- Right hypochondrium
- Cannot get above it
- Moves with respiration
- Dull to percussion.

Spleen

- Left hypochondrium
- Cannot get above it
- Moves with respiration
- Dull to percussion
- Has a notch.

Kidney

- Can get above it
- Doesn't move with respiration
- Resonant
- Ballotable.

EXAMINATION OF THE THYROID GLAND

Need a glass of water (may be beside the bed). Start by making general comments – does the child look well, do they seem appropriately grown?

Look

- Look from the front with the neck extended for enlargement of the thyroid gland
- Is the enlargement uniform or unilateral?
- Ask the child to take a drink – thyroid swelling should move upwards with swallowing
- Ask child to stick tongue out – a thyroglossal cyst will move upwards.

Palpate

- Palpate the gland whilst standing behind the child
- Assess size, shape consistency and surface of the mass
- Again ask to drink whilst palpating.

Also

- Palpate for lymphadenopathy
- Percuss sternum for retro-sternal extension
- Auscultate for bruits.

Scheme For Examination of Thyroid Status

- Look generally at the child; comment on growth
- Feel hands – warm and sweaty (hyperthyroid) or cold and blue (hypothyroid)
- Ask to hold arms outstretched for fine tremor (hyperthyroid)
- Count pulse – tachycardia (hyperthyroid), bradycardia (hypothyroid)
- Take blood pressure (wide pulse pressure in hyperthyroidism)

- Examine eyes for exophthalmos and lid lag (Grave's disease)
- Examine cardiovascular system for flow murmurs and hyperactive praecordium (hyperthyroidism)
- Examine abdomen for constipation (hypothyroid)
- Examine for a proximal myopathy (hyper or hypothyroidism)
- Pre-tibial oedema (hypothyroidism)
- Tendon reflexes (hypothyroidism – slow relaxation).

EXAMINATION OF A SHORT CHILD

Offer to plot height. Ask about previous heights. Ask about parental heights. Note pubertal status – may be obvious, eg post-pubertal girl.

1 Is the child obviously dysmorphic?

eg Turner's syndrome, Noonan's syndrome, Russell–Silver dwarfism, Prader–Willi syndrome. If yes, direct the examination towards that problem.

2 Does the child have a skeletal dysplasia?

eg achondroplasia, hypochondroplasia, spondyloepiphyseal dysplasia.

3 Is there an obvious systemic disease?

Thin child – eg cystic fibrosis/bronchiectasis, coeliac disease, inflammatory bowel disease.

Fat child – eg cushingoid, hypothyroidism, hypopituitarism/growth hormone deficiency.

4 Consider other possibilities

- Constitutional delay
- Familial short stature
- Emotional/food deprivation.

INTERPRETING PARENTAL HEIGHT

Expected centile = (mother's height centile + father's height centile)/2

Tall stature

Tall children and adolescents are frequently seen; remember the potential causes including familial tall stature, tall stature secondary to obesity and Marfan's syndrome.

Expected final adult height

BOY (father's height + [mother's height + 12.5 cm])/2

GIRL ([father's height – 12.5 cm] + mother's height)/2

EXAMINATION OF THE SKIN

This is difficult and it is not possible to have a scheme which is always applicable.

Aim for good exposure

- Look at the hands, nails and wrists
- Look at the elbows
- Exposure of other areas (front and back)
- Look at the child from head to toe including mouth and teeth
- If desperate ask if there is a rash and where it is
- Recognise common disorders.

Common Short Cases – Dermatology

Eczema

Strawberry naevus

Mongolian blue spot

Psoriasis

Capillary haemangioma

Café-au-lait spots (neurofibromatosis)

Sebaceous naevus

Vitiligo

Lipodystrophies

Molluscum contagiosum

Epidermolysis bullosa

Ectodermal dysplasia

Henoch–Schönlein purpura.

EXAMINATION OF THE JOINTS

Look

- General appearance of the child
- Any obvious clues, eg orthoses, shoes, splints
- Look for any deformity, erythema, swelling around the joint, scars from previous infection or surgery
- Look at muscle bulk
- Compare with normal joint.

Feel

- Watch patient's face while palpating the joint
- Feel for skin temperature, tenderness and joint effusion.

Move

Ask the child to move the joint before you move it to ensure that movement is not painful and to get some idea of the range of movement possible. It is important to do this as you don't want to cause pain as soon as you touch the patient!

Function

Assess the function of the joint if possible, eg ask the child to walk, pick up an object etc.

- Use one of the larger texts (Short cases for the Paediatric Membership, Beattie M, PasTest Ltd) to read about the examination of individual joints.

Common Short Cases – Rheumatology

Perthes' disease

Juvenile idiopathic (chronic) arthritis

Psoriatic arthritis

Juvenile dermatomyositis

Haemophilia

Osteogenesis imperfecta

Congenital dislocation of the hip

Toe walking

Hemihypertrophy.

DEVELOPMENTAL ASSESSMENT

Remember the areas of development

- Gross Motor
- Fine Motor and Vision
- Speech and Hearing
- Social.

In the assessment of a child's development in the exam it is essential to discuss milestones from each of these four areas.

MILESTONES

It is essential to know some of the developmental milestones. A selection of milestones is listed below.

6 WEEKS

Gross motor	holds chin up when prone, beginning to lose head lag
Fine motor and vision	follows object up to 180 degrees in the horizontal plane, watches people
Social	smiles

12 WEEKS (3 MONTHS)

Gross motor	lifts head and chest with extended arms when prone, reaches forward, but misses objects, supine early head control, loss of Moro reflex, makes defensive movements
Fine motor and vision	fixes and follows in the horizontal and vertical plane
Social	sustained social contact, listens to music, begins to vocalise

16 WEEKS (4 MONTHS)

Gross motor	lifts head and chest into vertical axis, legs extended, hands in midline, reaches and grasps objects and brings them to the mouth. No head lag on pulling to the sitting position. Held erect, pushes with feet
Social	laughs out loud, shows displeasure, excited at sight of food

28 WEEKS (7 MONTHS)

Gross motor	rolls over prone to supine (first) then supine to prone, sits with rounded back and leans forward on hands, supports most of weight on standing and bounces actively, reaches out and grasps for large objects
Fine motor and vision	transfers from hand to hand, grasps using radial grasp, rakes at pellets
Speech and hearing	polysyllabic vowel sounds formed
Social	prefers mother, babbles, enjoys mirror

40 WEEKS (9 MONTHS)

Gross motor	sits alone without support, back straight, pulls to standing position and cruises around the furniture, creeps and crawls
Fine motor and vision	grasps objects with thumb and forefinger, pokes at things with a forefinger, picks up a pellet with assisted pincer grip (using radial border of arm), uncovers hidden toy, object permanence
Speech and hearing	repetitive consonant sounds mama, dada, should pass distraction test (see later)
Social	responds to sound of name, plays peek-a-boo or pat-a-cake, waves bye-bye

1 YEAR

Gross motor	walks with one hand held, rises independently
Fine motor and vision	full pincer grip, releases objects on request
Speech and hearing	few words besides mama, dada, beginning to have meaning
Social	plays simple ball game, makes postural adjustments to dressing

15 MONTHS

Gross motor	walks alone, crawls upstairs
Fine motor and vision	makes tower of three cubes, makes line with crayon, inserts pellet into bottle
Speech and hearing	jargon, may name familiar objects
Social	hugs parents, indicates desires and needs

18 MONTHS

Gross motor	runs stiffly, sits on small chair, walks upstairs with hand held, explores
Fine motor and vision	tower of four cubes, imitates scribbling, imitates vertical strokes, dumps pellet
Speech and hearing	ten words, names pictures, identifies one or more body parts
Social	feeds self, seeks help, tells when wet/soiled, kisses parents with pucker

2 YEARS

Gross motor	runs well, walks up and down stairs one step at a time, opens doors, climbs on furniture, jumps
Fine motor and vision	tower of seven cubes, circular scribbling, imitates horizontal strokes
Speech and hearing	puts three words together (subject, verb, object)
Social	handles spoon well, listens to stories, tells immediate experiences, helps to undress

2 ½ YEARS

Gross motor	upstairs alternating feet
Fine motor and vision	tower of nine cubes, vertical and horizontal strokes but not yet a cross, forms closed figure
Speech and hearing	refers to self as I, uses proper name
Social	helps put things away, pretends in play

3 YEARS

Gross motor	rides tricycle, stands on one foot momentarily
Fine motor and vision	tower of ten cubes, imitates bridge of three cubes, copies circle, imitates cross
Speech and hearing	knows age and sex, counts three objects correctly, repeats three numbers
Social	plays simple games in parallel with other children, helps in dressing, washes hands

4 YEARS

Gross motor	hops on one foot, throws ball over hand, uses scissors to cut out picture, climbs well
Fine motor and vision	copies bridge from model, imitates construction of gate from five cubes, copies cross and square, draws a person with two to four parts without the head
Speech and hearing	counts four pennies accurately, tells a story
Social	plays with other children with beginning of social interaction, goes to toilet alone

5 YEARS

Gross motor	skips
Fine motor and vision	draws triangle from copy, names heavier of two weights
Speech and hearing	names four colours, repeats sentence of ten syllables, counts ten pennies correctly
Social	dresses and undresses, asks questions about the meaning of words, domestic role-playing

The ages given are for when you would expect 90% of children to have achieved the milestone stated. The ages above are the average ages to attain milestones. It is important to know the ages at which 90% of children would be expected to have achieved skills, as this may indicate further investigation if a child hasn't attained the skill by this age.

Common Short Cases – Child Development

It is essential to practise the assessment of development and the assessment of the special senses.

Think about the following scenarios and devise a plan for the assessment, incorporating the four areas of development (see above):

6 months old – Assess this infant's development

12 months old – Assess this infant's development

2 ½ years – Assess this child's development

Pre-school child – Assess this child's development

Assess this 2-year-old with delayed walking

Assess this 3-year-old who is not yet talking

Assess this 18-month-old whose parents are worried because he can't hear

Remember to use the College guidelines for assessment of hearing, assessment of vision and child health surveillance. Use one of the community paediatric text books for more information.

SCHEME FOR EXAMINATION OF THE CRANIAL NERVES

- Enquire about sense of smell, be prepared to examine formally if requested
- Test visual acuity
- Comment on any obvious abnormality such as squint and go on to examine formally if present
- Examine visual fields
- Examine eye movements
- Check for nystagmus – present at extremes of gaze
- Test the sensory divisions of the trigeminal nerve
- Test the motor component of the trigeminal nerve
- Test the facial nerve
- Test the auricular nerve grossly by asking the child if they can hear a very quiet noise that you make in each ear. Offer and know how to test formally
- The glossopharyngeal nerve can be tested by the gag reflex. This should not be attempted in the exam but do mention it.

  Remember that the gag reflex tests the glossopharyngeal (sensory) and vagal (motor) nerves. Ask the child to say 'ah' and look at the soft palate. A lesion of the vagus causes the palate on the contralateral side to be drawn upwards.
- Test the hypoglossal nerve by asking the patient to stick out their tongue and move it from side to side
- Test the accessory nerve by forced rotation of the head against resistance to check for sternomastoid weakness.

At the end of the examination you should ask to:

- Look at the fundi
- Assess pupillary responses to light and accommodation, offer to check corneal (V cranial nerve) and gag (IX cranial nerve) reflexes.

SCHEME FOR EXAMINATION OF THE EYES

- Look at the child for any obvious clues, eg squint, ptosis
- Does the child wear glasses?
- Look at the eyes – conjunctiva, pupils, lids
- Can the child see? Test both eyes – visual acuity
- Visual fields
- Eye movements
- Check for nystagmus
- Accommodation
- Pupil responses – direct and consensual light reflexes
- Cover test for squint
- Fundoscopy.

Squint is a commonly asked topic and it is important to go to an orthoptic clinic and revise the examination of squint and be confident about it.

Convex glasses correct long-sightedness

Long sight – difficulty with near vision

Concave glasses correct short-sightedness

Short sight – difficulty with distant vision

SCHEME FOR EXAMINATION OF THE PERIPHERAL MOTOR SYSTEM

Infants

Most of the information is gained by observation and so spend some time watching and playing with the infant. Try to get eye contact – see if the child will fix and follow in the horizontal and vertical planes. Look for any obvious dysmorphology. Assess spontaneous movement.

- Pull the child to sit – use one hand to pull up both hands and the other to support the head
- Hold the child by the trunk in the sitting position and assess standing posture
- Hold the child up prone looking at tone and head control
- Place the child on the bed prone to see if the child supports its head, supports itself on its forearms (3 months) or outstretched hands (6 months)
- Proceed with further examination depending on the initial findings Remember that if the head is extended when the child is held prone this may reflect extensor spasm and that head control is better assessed by pulling the child to sit.

Proceed to examine the tendon reflexes as you would in an older child.

Consider checking for primitive reflexes, eg Moro, asymmetric tonic neck reflex, grasp, etc if appropriate.

Older Children

Ask the child to walk first, unless there is an obvious reason why they can't (eg in a wheelchair).

- Look at muscle bulk, symmetry and for scars, eg tendo-Achilles shortening
- Examine tone – include testing for clonus
- Examine power
- Examine reflexes
- Further examination as appropriate.

Upper Motor Neurone or Lower Motor Neurone Lesions

Characteristics of an upper motor neurone lesion:

- Increased tone
- Clonus
- Reduced power
- Increased reflexes.

Characteristics of a lower motor neurone lesion:

- Wasting
- Reduced tone
- Fasciculation
- Reduced power
- Reduced reflexes.

EXAMINATION OF GAIT

Abnormalities to be looked for are:

- Hemiplegia
- Diplegia
- Ataxia
- Lower motor neurone problem
- Myopathy
- Orthopaedic problems/rheumatological disorders.

General points

First check with the child or parents that they can walk. Look at the child, do they look dysmorphic, is there an obvious cerebral palsy, is there a built up shoe, are there sticks or a wheelchair nearby?

Spastic gait

Ask the child to walk unaided – look at arm and leg movement for signs of hemiplegia. The arm will be flexed on the affected side. If you suspect hemiplegia ask the child to walk fast or walk on tip-toe, which will make the neurological disorder more pronounced. Continue looking – are the legs stiff and abducted? If so a diplegia is likely; a diplegia will also become more pronounced if you ask the child to walk fast or on tip-toe.

Ataxic gait

If the gait is not spastic the next thing to consider is whether it is ataxic (unsteady and broad based). Ask the child to heel-to-toe walk (you will need to demonstrate this). If the child is ataxic this will be difficult. Then ask the child to stand and to close their eyes. If the lesion is in the cerebellum there should be no deterioration. If the ataxia is as a consequence of a dorsal column problem the child will fall (Romberg's sign).

Neuromuscular problem

The next possibility is that you are dealing with either a neuromuscular or a lower motor neurone problem. Look for a waddling gait and foot drop. Examine for Gower's sign.

Others

Consider either an orthopaedic or a rheumatological problem.

SCHEME FOR CEREBELLAR EXAMINATION

- Test eye movements and look for nystagmus – horizontal and maximal looking to the side of the lesion
- Ask the child a question and listen for dysarthria
- Test co-ordination. Ask the child to touch his/her finger and then your nose with his/her index finger. Look for past pointing or intention tremor. Assess rapidly alternating movements (dysdiadochokinesia)
- Examine the arms and legs for hypotonia and hyporeflexia
- Ask the child to sit to check for truncal ataxia
- Stand the child up and examine for Romberg's sign to differentiate dorsal column from cerebellar disease
- Think of the causes of ataxia and look for associated signs, eg telangiectasia (ataxia telangiectasia) or pes cavus (Friedreich's ataxia).

Common Short Cases – Neurology

Cerebral palsy

- Hemiplegia
- Diplegia
- Quadriplegia
- Ataxic
- Athetoid.

Neuromuscular disease (older child)

- Duchenne muscular dystrophy
- Kugelberg–Welander disease
- Dermatomyositis
- Peroneal muscular atrophy.

The floppy infant

- Werdnig–Hoffman disease
- Myotonic dystrophy
- Down's syndrome
- Failure to thrive.

Spina bifida

Ataxia

- Friedreich's ataxia
- Ataxia telangiectasia
- Ataxic cerebral palsy.

Neurocutaneous syndromes

- Neurofibromatosis
- Tuberous sclerosis
- Sturge–Weber syndrome.

INDEX

PASTEST – DEDICATED TO YOUR SUCCESS

PasTest has been publishing books for medical students and doctors for over 30 years. Our extensive experience means that we are always one step ahead when it comes to knowledge of current trends in Paediatric exams.

We use only the best authors, which enables us to tailor our books to meet your revision needs. We incorporate feedback from candidates to ensure that our books are continually improved.

This commitment to quality ensures that candidates who buy PasTest books achieve successful exam results.

Delivery to your door

With a busy lifestyle, nobody enjoys walking to the shops for something that may or may not be in stock. Let us take the hassle and deliver direct to your door. We will dispatch your book within 24 hours of receiving your order.

How to Order:

www.pastest.co.uk
To order books safely and securely online, shop at our website.

Telephone: +44 (0)1565 752000 Fax: +44 (0)1565 650264
For priority mail order and have your credit card to hand when you call.

Write to us at:
PasTest Ltd
FREEPOST
Haig Road
Parkgate Industrial Estate
Knutsford
WA16 7BR